BREAST CANCER

From Diagnosis to Breakthrough Treatments: Everything You Need to Know

Dr. Sophie Domingues-Montanari

Disclaimer

The author has undertaken extensive research and due diligence to provide accurate, up-to-date information in this book. However, the rapidly evolving field of cancer research, alongside individual variations in health conditions and responses, means that some information may become outdated or may not apply universally to all readers. Therefore, it is imperative that readers exercise their own discretion and critical thinking when interpreting and implementing the concepts presented herein.

This book is not intended to serve as a substitute for professional medical advice, diagnosis, or treatment. Readers are strongly encouraged to consult with qualified healthcare professionals, including oncologists, nutritionists, or other relevant specialists, before making any changes to their health regimen, particularly in relation to fasting, cancer treatment, or dietary modifications. Individual health circumstances can vary widely, and what may be beneficial for one person may not be appropriate for another.

The author expressly disclaims any responsibility for adverse effects or consequences resulting from the use or application of the information provided in this book. This includes, but is not limited to, any potential losses, injuries, or damages— whether direct, indirect, incidental, consequential, or punitive—that may arise from reliance on this material.

By choosing to read this book and apply any of its contents, readers acknowledge their understanding of this disclaimer and agree to indemnify and hold harmless the author, as well as any affiliated parties, from any and all claims, demands, or liabilities arising from the use of the information contained herein. The information in this book reflects the author's personal views and is not necessarily indicative of the consensus within the medical community. Readers are encouraged to seek a variety of perspectives and information to make informed decisions regarding their health and wellness.

Copyright Statement

Copyright © Sophie Domingues-Montanari, 2025. All rights reserved.

This publication is protected by international copyright laws and treaties. No part of this work may be reproduced, distributed, or transmitted in any form or by any means—whether electronic, mechanical, photocopying, recording, or otherwise—without the explicit prior written consent of the author, Sophie Domingues-Montanari. This includes, but is not limited to, copying, adaptation, modification, or translation of any part of this book.

You may, however, make brief quotations for the purposes of criticism, comment, or educational use, provided that such use falls within the bounds of fair use as defined by copyright law and is properly attributed to the author.

Unauthorized reproduction or distribution of any part of this publication may result in severe civil and criminal penalties, and will be vigorously pursued by the author and publisher.

Table of Contents

BREAST CANCER 5

Disclaimer 7

Copyright Statement 9

Table of Contents 11

Introduction 15
   Overview of the Book 15
   Breast Cancer Statistics 16

Chapter 1: Understanding Breast Cancer 19
   What is Breast Cancer? 19
   Types of Breast Cancer 20
   Risk Factors 23
   Myths vs. Facts 27

Chapter 2: The Biology of Breast Cancer 31
   Tumor Development 31
   Molecular Subtypes 35
   Genetic Mutations 39

Chapter 3: Prevention and Risk Reduction 45
   Lifestyle Factors 45
   Breastfeeding 49
   Hormonal Therapy 52
   Environmental Factors 56

Chapter 4: Early Detection and Diagnosis 63
   Screening Methods 63
   Self-Examination 68
   Signs and Symptoms 72
   The Diagnostic Process 76

Chapter 5: Staging and Prognosis 83
   Understanding Breast Cancer Staging 83

Lymph Node Involvement 88
　　Prognostic Factors 92
　　The Role of Molecular Testing 97

Chapter 6: Treatment Options 103
　　Surgery 103
　　Radiation Therapy 108
　　Chemotherapy 113
　　Targeted Therapies 119
　　Immunotherapy 123
　　Hormone Therapy 127
　　Clinical Trials 132

Chapter 7: Coping with the Diagnosis 139
　　Emotional and Psychological Impact 139
　　Support Systems 143
　　Mental Health Resources 147
　　Life After Treatment 152

Chapter 8: Nutrition and Lifestyle During Treatment 157
　　Dietary Considerations 157
　　Exercise 161
　　Supplements 166
　　Weight Management, Diet, and Fasting 170

Chapter 9: The Latest Advances in Research 175
　　Personalized Medicine 175
　　Immunotherapy Breakthroughs 179
　　Targeted Therapies 184
　　Early Detection Innovations 189
　　Preventive Treatments 193

Chapter 10: Living with Breast Cancer 199
　　Survivorship 199
　　Long-Term Follow-Up 204
　　Quality of Life 208
　　Seeking Financial Support 213
　　Legal and Financial Considerations 219

Chapter 11: Supporting a Loved One with Breast Cancer *227*
   How to Be There for Someone 227
   Understanding the Treatment Process......................232
   Caring for the Caregiver...237

Conclusion *243*
   Key Takeaways 243
   Hope and Future Outlook..250
   Glossary of Medical Terms 252
   Frequently Asked Questions (FAQs) 257
   Resources for Information and Support....................264

Introduction

Overview of the Book

Breast Cancer is one of the most common and impactful diseases affecting millions worldwide. Whether you are a patient navigating your own breast cancer journey, a family member or friend seeking ways to support a loved one, or a student of medicine or science, this guide is here to offer clarity, knowledge, and a deeper understanding.

This book delves into:

- **The basics**: What breast cancer is, how it develops, and the different types.

- **Risk factors**: Genetic, environmental, and lifestyle influences that can increase the risk of breast cancer.

- **Diagnosis and staging**: From screening techniques to the diagnostic process, we explore how doctors determine the presence, stage, and severity of cancer.

- **Treatment options**: A detailed overview of the treatments available, including surgery, chemotherapy, radiation, immunotherapy, and newer targeted therapies.

- **Emotional support and survivorship**: Understanding the emotional impact of a breast cancer diagnosis, managing mental health, and living a fulfilling life post-treatment.

- **Latest advances**: Cutting-edge research in prevention, treatment, and personalized medicine that offers hope for the future.

The goal of this book is not just to inform, but to empower. Whether you are dealing with a recent diagnosis, supporting a loved one, or simply interested in understanding the disease, this guide is meant to be a trusted source of information and support. Every chapter has been designed to walk you through every stage of breast cancer—from understanding its biological roots to navigating treatment and recovery.

Breast Cancer Statistics

Breast cancer is a leading global health issue, impacting millions of lives every year. Its prevalence makes it a key focus for both public health initiatives and ongoing research. Understanding the statistics surrounding breast cancer can underscore the importance of awareness, early detection, and the need for continued advancements in treatment.

- **Incidence**: According to the World Health Organization (WHO), breast cancer is the most common cancer worldwide, accounting for nearly **25% of all new cancer cases** in women. In 2020, there were **2.3 million new cases** diagnosed globally.

- **Mortality**: Breast cancer is also the leading cause of cancer-related deaths in women worldwide. In 2020, approximately **685,000 women** died from breast cancer, which represents **15% of all cancer deaths**.

- **Survival Rates**: The survival rate for breast cancer varies by region, stage at diagnosis, and access to treatment. However, the **5-year survival rate** for breast cancer has improved significantly over the last few decades, now exceeding **90%** in high-income countries for localized stages.

- **Geographic Disparities**: Rates of breast cancer are higher in developed countries, likely due to better detection and reporting. However, survival outcomes tend to be worse in low- and middle-income countries due to challenges such as late diagnosis, lack of treatment facilities, and financial barriers.

The prevalence of breast cancer emphasizes the need for widespread awareness campaigns. Early detection through regular screenings, self-exams, and awareness of symptoms can lead to earlier diagnoses and better outcomes. Regular mammograms and breast exams are crucial for catching the disease early. In the U.S., **women aged 40 and older** are generally recommended to have annual mammograms, although individual guidelines may vary depending on family history and other factors. Modern treatment protocols, including surgery, chemotherapy, targeted therapies, immunotherapy, and hormone therapy, have dramatically improved survival rates. However, the treatment plan for each individual is increasingly personalized, based on factors such as the molecular subtype of the cancer and genetic testing results.

Chapter 1: Understanding Breast Cancer

What is Breast Cancer?

Breast cancer is a disease that starts in the cells of the breast. Like all cancers, it begins when normal cells in the body start growing out of control. In the case of breast cancer, this growth happens in the cells of the breast tissue, which can spread to other parts of the body if left untreated.

The breast is made up of different parts, including the **lobules** (the milk-producing glands), **ducts** (the tubes that carry milk to the nipple), and connective tissue. Breast cancer most often starts in either the lobules or the ducts. When cancer starts in the ducts, it's called **ductal carcinoma**, and when it starts in the lobules, it's called **lobular carcinoma**.

The cells in the breast may change in a variety of ways, but the most important sign that something is wrong is that these cells start growing uncontrollably. Normally, cells in our body grow, divide, and die in a regular cycle. But when this cycle is disrupted—either because the cells don't die when they should or because they divide too rapidly—cancer can develop.

What makes breast cancer even trickier is that not all cells behave the same way. Some cancers grow slowly, while others spread quickly. These cancer cells can break away from the original tumor, travel through the bloodstream or lymphatic system, and spread to other parts of the body. This is known as **metastasis**, and it's why early detection and treatment are so important.

Breast cancer is often **silent in its early stages**—meaning there may be no obvious signs or symptoms. That's why regular screenings and paying attention to any changes in your body, like lumps or pain in the breast, are so important. The good news is that, with early diagnosis and treatment, many people go on to live long, healthy lives.

Types of Breast Cancer

Breast cancer isn't just one disease—it's actually a group of diseases, and the type of breast cancer a person has depends on where it starts and how it behaves. Let's explore the main types of breast cancer you might hear about.

Invasive Ductal Carcinoma (IDC)

This is the **most common type of breast cancer**, making up about 70-80% of all cases. IDC begins in the **milk ducts** of the breast, which are responsible for carrying milk to the nipple. Over time, the cancer spreads beyond the ducts into the surrounding tissue. Because it can spread to other parts of the body, IDC is considered an "invasive" cancer. The good news is that, because it's so common, there are plenty of treatments and a lot of research focused on this type.

Invasive Lobular Carcinoma (ILC)

ILC starts in the **lobules** of the breast, which are the glands that produce milk. Like IDC, this type can also spread to other parts of the body, so it's classified as invasive. ILC accounts for about 10-15% of all breast cancer cases. It can be a little trickier to detect on a mammogram or ultrasound because it often doesn't form a lump but instead spreads out in thin layers of tissue. Despite that, many people with ILC can still be successfully treated.

Ductal Carcinoma in Situ (DCIS)

DCIS is a **non-invasive** or "pre-cancerous" condition where abnormal cells are found in the milk ducts but have not yet spread to surrounding tissue. It's sometimes referred to as stage 0 breast cancer. Though DCIS isn't life-threatening on its own, it can sometimes lead to invasive cancer if not treated. The good news is that most people diagnosed with DCIS are successfully treated, often with surgery or radiation.

Lobular Carcinoma in Situ (LCIS)

LCIS is another **non-invasive** condition where abnormal cells are found in the lobules of the breast but have not spread to other parts of the breast tissue. Although LCIS isn't technically cancer, it can increase the risk of developing invasive breast cancer in the future. People with LCIS are often closely monitored with regular screenings.

Inflammatory Breast Cancer (IBC)

IBC is a **rare** but aggressive form of breast cancer. Unlike other types, IBC doesn't usually form a lump. Instead, the skin of the breast becomes red, swollen, and warm, giving the appearance of inflammation (hence the name). IBC tends to spread more quickly and is often diagnosed at a later stage. While it's more difficult to treat than some other types of breast cancer, there are still treatments that can be effective, and many people with IBC go on to live long lives with the right care.

Triple-Negative Breast Cancer (TNBC)

Triple-negative breast cancer is a more **aggressive** type of breast cancer that doesn't have three common receptors that are often found in breast cancer cells—estrogen receptors, progesterone receptors, and HER2. This means that treatments like hormone therapy and HER2-targeted therapies won't be effective. Although it tends to grow and spread more quickly than other types, TNBC can sometimes be treated with chemotherapy and immunotherapy, and researchers are working on new targeted therapies to improve outcomes.

HER2-Positive Breast Cancer

HER2-positive breast cancer happens when there are **too many copies of the HER2 gene** in the breast cancer cells, causing the cancer cells to grow and divide more quickly. About 15-20% of breast cancers are HER2-positive. Fortunately, HER2-positive breast cancer can be treated with **targeted therapies** like Herceptin, which specifically targets the HER2 protein to slow down the growth of the cancer.

Paget's Disease of the Nipple

Paget's disease is a **rare form** of breast cancer that affects the skin of the nipple and the areola (the dark circle around the nipple). It often starts with itching, redness, or flaking skin on the nipple, sometimes mistaken for a skin condition. Paget's disease is usually associated with either IDC or ILC, and treatment typically involves surgery, sometimes along with radiation or chemotherapy.

Each type of breast cancer behaves differently, which is why doctors tailor treatment based on the specific type and other factors, like the size of the tumor and whether the cancer has spread.

Risk Factors

Breast cancer, like many other diseases, is influenced by a variety of **risk factors**—things that can increase the likelihood of developing the disease. These factors can be **genetic**, **hormonal**, **environmental**, or related to **lifestyle** choices. Let's take a closer look at each of these to understand how they contribute to the risk of breast cancer.

Genetic Factors (BRCA1 and BRCA2)

Some people have a higher risk of breast cancer due to **genetic mutations** passed down from their parents. The **BRCA1** and **BRCA2** genes are the most well-known genetic risk factors. These genes help repair damaged DNA, but when they are mutated, they can fail to do their job properly, increasing the risk of breast and ovarian cancers.

- **BRCA1** mutations are linked to a higher risk of both breast and ovarian cancer.
- **BRCA2** mutations also increase the risk of breast cancer, but the risk is somewhat lower than for BRCA1.

People with these mutations may develop cancer at a younger age, and the cancer may also be more aggressive. If you have a family history of breast or ovarian cancer, especially in several close relatives, genetic testing may help assess your risk.

Hormonal Factors

Hormones, particularly **estrogen** and **progesterone**, play a significant role in the development of breast cancer. These hormones can fuel the growth of some types of breast cancer, especially those that are **hormone receptor-positive** (which means the cancer cells have receptors for estrogen and/or progesterone). Here are some hormonal factors that can influence risk:

- **Early Menstruation**: If a woman started menstruating at an early age (before 12), her exposure to estrogen over her lifetime is longer, which may increase her risk.

- **Late Menopause**: Similarly, if a woman experiences menopause after age 55, her body is exposed to estrogen for a longer period, which can raise her risk.

- **Pregnancy and Breastfeeding**: Having children later in life or not having children at all may increase the risk. On the flip side, **breastfeeding** can slightly reduce the risk of breast cancer.

- **Hormone Replacement Therapy (HRT)**: Using hormone replacement therapy, especially combined estrogen and progesterone, for an extended period after menopause has been shown to increase the risk of breast cancer. The longer someone uses HRT, the higher their risk.

Environmental Factors

There are certain **environmental exposures** that can increase the risk of breast cancer. While these factors are harder to control, being aware of them can help you take steps to limit your exposure:

- **Radiation Exposure**: If you've had significant exposure to radiation, such as through radiation therapy to the chest for another type of cancer, your risk of breast cancer may be higher. This risk is particularly relevant if the radiation occurred during adolescence or early adulthood when breast tissue is still developing.

- **Environmental Chemicals**: Some chemicals in the environment, like **pesticides** and **pollutants**, have been linked to breast cancer risk. Though research is ongoing, certain industrial chemicals, like those found in plastics (such as BPA), may play a role in increasing risk, particularly in younger women.

Lifestyle Factors

Certain lifestyle choices can either increase or decrease the risk of breast cancer. Making healthier choices can have a significant impact on your overall health, including reducing the risk of developing breast cancer:

- **Alcohol Consumption**: Drinking alcohol is associated with an increased risk of breast cancer. The more alcohol consumed, the higher the risk. Studies suggest that alcohol can increase estrogen levels, which may fuel the growth of some types of breast cancer.

- **Physical Inactivity**: Lack of exercise is linked to a higher risk of breast cancer. Regular physical activity helps maintain a healthy weight, reduce estrogen levels, and improve overall health, all of which can lower breast cancer risk.

- **Obesity**: Being overweight or obese, especially after menopause, can increase the risk of breast cancer. This is partly because fat tissue produces extra estrogen, which may promote the growth of hormone-receptor-positive breast cancers.

- **Diet**: While no single food can prevent or cause breast cancer, a diet high in processed foods and unhealthy fats can contribute to weight gain and obesity, which can increase risk. On the other hand, a diet rich in fruits, vegetables, whole grains, and healthy fats may help lower your risk.

- **Smoking**: Smoking is associated with an increased risk of several cancers, including breast cancer, particularly in premenopausal women. Chemicals in tobacco can damage DNA in breast cells, leading to cancer.

Other Factors

- **Age**: The older you get, the higher your risk of developing breast cancer. Most breast cancers are diagnosed in women over the age of 50, though it can affect younger women as well.

- **Family History**: Having close relatives (mother, sister, daughter) with breast cancer increases your risk. However, 85% of breast cancer cases occur in women with no family history of the disease, so it's important not to rely solely on family history for risk assessment.

- **Personal History**: If you've already had breast cancer in one breast, you're at a higher risk of developing it in the other breast or having a recurrence in the same breast.

- **Race and Ethnicity**: Some racial and ethnic groups have higher rates of breast cancer than others. For instance, white women have a higher risk of developing breast cancer compared to African American women, though African American women are more likely to be diagnosed at a younger age and with more aggressive forms of the disease.

Understanding your risk factors is crucial in taking steps toward prevention, early detection, and treatment. While some factors are out of our control (like genetics and age), many others—such as lifestyle choices and environmental exposures—can be managed to help reduce your risk. Regular screenings, staying active, eating well, and making healthier choices can all contribute to lowering your breast cancer risk and improving your overall health.

Myths vs. Facts

There are many **myths and misconceptions** about breast cancer that can confuse and mislead people. Let's clear up some of the most common myths and replace them with the facts, so you can be more informed and better equipped to handle your health decisions.

Myth 1: Breast cancer only affects older women.

Fact: While breast cancer is more common in women over the age of 50, **younger women** can also develop it. In fact, about 1 in 8 breast cancer cases occur in women under the age of 45. The risk increases with age, but age alone is not the only factor. Regular screenings are important, even for women in their 20s and 30s, especially if they have other risk factors like a family history of breast cancer.

Myth 2: If you don't have a family history of breast cancer, you're not at risk.

Fact: Most women with breast cancer do not have a family history of the disease. In fact, around 85% of breast cancer cases occur in women with no family history of the disease. While family history can increase your risk, other factors, like hormonal, lifestyle, and environmental influences, play a major role too. It's important to be proactive with breast health regardless of your family history.

Myth 3: A breast lump always means cancer.

Fact: Not all lumps in the breast are cancerous. In fact, many women have lumps in their breasts that are benign (non-cancerous), such as cysts or fibrocystic changes. However, any new lump or change in the breast should still be evaluated by a doctor, as only a medical professional can determine whether it's something to be concerned about. Early detection is key, but remember that not every lump is cause for alarm.

Myth 4: Deodorant or antiperspirant causes breast cancer.

Fact: There is **no scientific evidence** linking deodorants or antiperspirants to breast cancer. This myth likely originated from concerns about aluminum compounds found in some antiperspirants, but studies have not shown that these ingredients cause cancer. Breast cancer typically begins in the ducts or lobules of the breast, areas far from where deodorant or antiperspirant would be applied.

Myth 5: Wearing a bra can cause breast cancer.

Fact: There is **no proven link** between wearing a bra and the development of breast cancer. Some studies have suggested that tight-fitting bras could cause issues with lymphatic drainage, but there is no scientific evidence to support the idea that wearing a bra, underwire or not, increases the risk of breast cancer. This is another myth with no factual basis.

Myth 6: Mastectomy guarantees that breast cancer won't come back.

Fact: While **mastectomy** (surgical removal of one or both breasts) can significantly reduce the risk of breast cancer recurring in the breast tissue, it **does not eliminate the risk entirely**. Breast cancer can spread to other parts of the body, such as the lymph nodes, liver, or lungs. This is why doctors often recommend additional treatments like chemotherapy, radiation, or hormone therapy, even after a mastectomy, to lower the risk of recurrence.

Myth 7: Only women get breast cancer.

Fact: While breast cancer is far more common in women, **men can get breast cancer too**. Although the risk is much lower in men (about 1 in 1,000), it does happen. Men have a small amount of breast tissue, and cancer can develop there. Because men aren't generally aware of the risk, they may not recognize symptoms, leading to delayed diagnosis. It's important for everyone, regardless of gender, to be aware of the signs and symptoms of breast cancer.

Myth 8: If you have a mammogram and it's clear, you don't need to worry.

Fact: While mammograms are an essential tool for detecting breast cancer early, **no screening method is 100% foolproof**. Mammograms can miss some cancers, particularly in dense breast tissue. Other screening options, like ultrasound or MRI, may be recommended if you have dense breasts or other risk factors. It's important to talk to your doctor about your individual screening needs.

Myth 9: Chemotherapy is the only treatment for breast cancer.

Fact: Chemotherapy is one of the treatments used for breast cancer, but it is not the only option. Treatment plans are personalized and may include a combination of **surgery, radiation therapy, hormone therapy, targeted therapy, and chemotherapy** depending on the type and stage of breast cancer. New treatments are constantly being researched, and many of these are less invasive and have fewer side effects than traditional chemotherapy.

Myth 10: If you're diagnosed with breast cancer, there's nothing you can do.

Fact: A breast cancer diagnosis can feel overwhelming, but there are **many treatment options** and **support systems** available. Survival rates have significantly improved in recent years, thanks to early detection, better treatments, and advancements in research. With the right treatment, many people with breast cancer live long, healthy lives. It's also important to remember that support—whether emotional, physical, or through a strong healthcare team—can make a big difference.

It's important to challenge myths and misconceptions about breast cancer to reduce fear and encourage informed decisions. By understanding the facts, you'll be better equipped to take control of your health and make choices that are right for you. Regular screenings, a healthy lifestyle, and open communication with your healthcare provider are key to breast cancer awareness and prevention.

Chapter 2: The Biology of Breast Cancer

Tumor Development

Breast cancer, like all cancers, begins when **normal cells** in the body start to behave abnormally. This process, known as **tumor development**, involves a series of stages where cells grow uncontrollably, and may spread to other parts of the body. Understanding this process helps explain why cancer can be so dangerous and how it can affect various organs.

The Formation of Tumors

At the start of breast cancer development, **normal cells** in the breast tissue undergo genetic changes, known as **mutations**. These mutations can occur for several reasons: exposure to harmful chemicals, radiation, inherited genetic mutations, or just random cellular errors. When these cells start to divide and multiply uncontrollably, they form a **tumor**—a mass of abnormal tissue.

There are two main types of tumors:

- **Benign Tumors**: These are non-cancerous growths. While they may grow and push against surrounding tissues, they do not spread to other parts of the body. In the case of benign breast conditions, such as cysts or fibroadenomas, they are typically not a threat.

- **Malignant Tumors**: These are **cancerous tumors**. Malignant cells can invade nearby tissues and spread to other parts of the body through a process called **metastasis**.

How Cancerous Cells Grow

Once a tumor is formed, the cancerous cells continue to grow and divide at an accelerated rate. Unlike normal cells, which have a lifespan and are programmed to die when they are no longer needed (a process called **apoptosis**), cancer cells evade this mechanism and keep growing.

This abnormal growth is driven by several factors:

- **Genetic mutations**: Mutations in genes responsible for controlling cell division and repair can cause cancer cells to proliferate uncontrollably.

- **Angiogenesis**: To support their rapid growth, cancer cells need nutrients and oxygen. To get this, they can stimulate the growth of new blood vessels, a process known as **angiogenesis**. These new blood vessels supply the tumor with the nutrients it needs to continue growing.

- **Increased survival**: Cancer cells often develop mechanisms that help them avoid the body's immune system, allowing them to survive longer than normal cells.

Invasion: Cancer Spreads to Nearby Tissues

As cancer cells grow, they can invade the surrounding healthy tissues. This is called **local invasion**. The cancerous cells break through the **basement membrane**, a thin layer that normally keeps cells in place. They then move into the surrounding tissues, including muscles, lymph nodes, and other structures within the breast.

The ability of cancer cells to invade and infiltrate nearby tissues makes them more dangerous and harder to treat. This is why **early detection** of breast cancer is crucial—catching it before it invades other areas of the body can improve treatment outcomes.

Metastasis: The Spread of Cancer

One of the most alarming features of cancer is its ability to **metastasize**—to spread from its original site to other parts of the body. Cancer cells can travel through the bloodstream or lymphatic system (a network of vessels and nodes that help fight infection). Here's how metastasis works:

- **Lymphatic Spread**: The lymphatic system is one of the primary routes through which breast cancer spreads. If the cancer cells enter the **lymphatic vessels**, they can travel to nearby **lymph nodes**, which are small, bean-shaped structures that help filter harmful substances. **Lymph nodes** in the armpit (axillary nodes) are often the first to be affected in breast cancer, which is why doctors check them during physical exams and biopsies.

- **Bloodstream Spread**: Cancer cells can also enter the bloodstream, allowing them to travel to distant organs such as the **liver, lungs, bones**, or even the **brain**. This is known as **hematogenous spread**. Once the cancer cells reach these distant organs, they can form secondary tumors, which are known as **metastases**.

Cancer that has spread to other parts of the body is harder to treat and can require more aggressive treatment, such as **chemotherapy**, **targeted therapy**, or **immunotherapy**.

Staging of Cancer

The stage of breast cancer refers to how far the cancer has spread. It is an essential part of diagnosing the disease and determining the treatment plan. The most common staging system used is the **TNM system**, which considers:

- **T (Tumor size)**: How large the primary tumor is.
- **N (Nodes)**: Whether cancer has spread to nearby lymph nodes.
- **M (Metastasis)**: Whether the cancer has spread to other organs or distant parts of the body.

The stage of the cancer is described using numbers from **0 to IV**, with **Stage 0** being localized (non-invasive), and **Stage IV** indicating metastatic cancer, where cancer has spread beyond the breast.

The Role of Hormones in Cancer Spread

Some breast cancers are **hormone receptor-positive**, meaning they rely on hormones like **estrogen** and **progesterone** to fuel their growth. These cancers are more likely to grow quickly and may have a higher chance of spreading (metastasizing). Hormone therapy, which blocks the effects of these hormones, is often used to treat these types of breast cancer.

Why Tumor Growth and Spread Matter

The growth and spread of tumors are why breast cancer can be so dangerous. As the cancer grows, it takes up space, destroys healthy tissues, and interferes with normal bodily functions. When it spreads to other parts of the body, it can affect vital organs like the liver, lungs, and bones, leading to complications that can be life-threatening.

However, not all breast cancers spread quickly. Some types are slow-growing and may stay confined to the breast tissue for a long time. This is why early detection is key—cancers that are caught before they metastasize are often easier to treat and have better outcomes.

Molecular Subtypes

Breast cancer is not a one-size-fits-all disease. While the **lump in the breast** might look similar, the biology behind it can vary greatly from person to person. This variation is why breast cancer is often classified into **molecular subtypes** based on the **genetic makeup** and **behavior** of the cancer cells. Understanding these subtypes is crucial because it influences treatment decisions and helps predict how the cancer will behave.

There are **five major molecular subtypes** of breast cancer. These subtypes are primarily defined by the presence or absence of specific receptors on the surface of cancer cells. Let's explore them in more detail:

Hormone Receptor-Positive (HR-positive)

This is one of the most common types of breast cancer. In **HR-positive breast cancer**, the cancer cells have receptors for **estrogen** and/or **progesterone**, two hormones that can fuel the growth of the cancer. When these hormones bind to the receptors on the surface of cancer cells, they trigger the growth and multiplication of the cancerous cells.

- **What this means**: Hormone receptor-positive cancers tend to grow more slowly than other types of breast cancer, and they are often more treatable. **Hormone therapy** (such as **tamoxifen** or **aromatase inhibitors**) is often used to block the effect of these hormones, either by blocking the receptor or lowering the levels of estrogen and progesterone in the body.

- **How common is it?**: Around **70-80%** of all breast cancers are hormone receptor-positive.

HER2-Positive (Human Epidermal Growth Factor Receptor 2)

HER2 is a protein found on the surface of some cancer cells. When the **HER2 gene** is amplified (increased copies of the gene), it leads to an overproduction of the HER2 protein, making the cancer cells grow and divide more quickly. This type of breast cancer is known as **HER2-positive**.

- **What this means**: HER2-positive cancers are **aggressive** and tend to grow faster than hormone receptor-positive cancers. However, they are also **treatable** with targeted therapies that specifically target the HER2 protein. **Trastuzumab** (Herceptin) and **pertuzumab** (Perjeta) are examples of drugs that target HER2, and they can significantly improve outcomes for patients with HER2-positive breast cancer.
- **How common is it?**: About **20-25%** of breast cancers are HER2-positive.

Triple-Negative Breast Cancer (TNBC)

This type of breast cancer is **negative** for the three most common markers: **estrogen receptors (ER)**, **progesterone receptors (PR)**, and **HER2**. In other words, **triple-negative** breast cancer does not have receptors for estrogen or progesterone and is not driven by the HER2 protein.

- **What this means**: Triple-negative breast cancer tends to be more **aggressive** and has fewer targeted treatment options. Since it doesn't respond to hormone therapy or HER2-targeted treatments,

chemotherapy is often the main treatment for this type of breast cancer. However, recent advancements in **immunotherapy** and **PARP inhibitors** are providing new treatment options, especially for patients with genetic mutations like **BRCA1** or **BRCA2**.

- **How common is it?**: Triple-negative breast cancer accounts for about **10-15%** of all breast cancers, and it is more common in **younger women**, **African American women**, and those with a **BRCA1 mutation**.

Luminal A and Luminal B (Subtypes of Hormone Receptor-Positive)

These two subtypes are part of the broader category of **hormone receptor-positive** cancers but differ in their **biological characteristics** and **prognosis**.

- **Luminal A**:
    - **What it is**: This is a **less aggressive** subtype of hormone receptor-positive breast cancer. It has low levels of **HER2** and **Ki-67** (a protein that indicates how fast the cancer cells are dividing).
    - **What this means**: Luminal A cancers tend to have a **better prognosis** and are more likely to respond well to **hormone therapy** alone.
    - **How common is it?**: Luminal A is the most common subtype of breast cancer, making up about **50-60%** of all breast cancer cases.
- **Luminal B**:

- **What it is**: Luminal B is similar to Luminal A but is often more **aggressive**, with **higher levels of HER2** or **Ki-67**. It can also grow more quickly.
- **What this means**: Luminal B cancers may require additional treatments, such as **chemotherapy** or **HER2-targeted therapies**, along with hormone therapy.
- **How common is it?**: Luminal B makes up about **10-20%** of breast cancers and is more likely to occur in **younger women** or those who are **pre-menopausal**.

Basal-like Breast Cancer

Basal-like breast cancer is often referred to as a **subtype of triple-negative breast cancer**, but it has some distinct features. These cancers have characteristics similar to the **basal cells** of the breast, which are cells that line the ducts and lobules.

- **What this means**: Basal-like breast cancer tends to be **aggressive**, with a higher likelihood of spreading. It does not respond to hormone therapy or HER2-targeted treatments, so treatment typically focuses on chemotherapy. Recent studies suggest that **immunotherapy** may offer promise for some patients with this subtype.
- **How common is it?**: This subtype is a part of **triple-negative breast cancer**, so it makes up around **10-15%** of all breast cancers.

Why Molecular Subtypes Matter

Understanding the molecular subtype of breast cancer is crucial because it helps doctors determine the most effective treatment plan. Some subtypes respond well to hormone therapy, while others require chemotherapy, targeted therapies, or a combination of approaches. **Genetic testing**, such as the **Oncotype DX** test, can help determine the likelihood of recurrence and guide treatment choices for hormone receptor-positive cancers.

Each subtype also varies in its **prognosis** and the **likelihood of metastasis**. By identifying the subtype early, doctors can tailor the treatment to the specific characteristics of the cancer, improving outcomes and minimizing unnecessary treatments.

Genetic Mutations

Breast cancer doesn't just happen by chance; sometimes, it can be linked to **genetic mutations** passed down through families. These mutations can significantly increase a person's risk of developing breast cancer. The most well-known mutations associated with breast cancer are **BRCA1** and **BRCA2**, but other genetic factors also play a role. Understanding these genetic mutations helps us better understand why some people are at higher risk and how they can take proactive steps for early detection and prevention.

What Are Genetic Mutations?

A **genetic mutation** is a change or alteration in the DNA sequence. Our DNA contains the instructions for how our cells function, grow, and divide. Normally, cells divide and grow in a controlled way, but mutations can disrupt this process, leading to uncontrolled cell growth, which is how cancer forms. While some mutations occur randomly due to environmental factors or aging, others are inherited from one's parents and are present in a person's DNA from birth.

In the case of **breast cancer**, certain inherited mutations increase the risk of developing the disease. These mutations are typically found in genes that are responsible for **repairing DNA damage**, regulating cell growth, or controlling the death of abnormal cells.

The BRCA1 and BRCA2 Mutations

The **BRCA1** and **BRCA2** genes are the most famous **tumor suppressor genes** involved in breast cancer. These genes are responsible for producing proteins that help repair damaged DNA and maintain the stability of the cell's genetic material. When these genes are mutated, they can no longer perform their repair function effectively, leading to an accumulation of genetic errors that may result in cancer.

- **BRCA1 Mutation**: Women with a **BRCA1 mutation** have a significantly increased risk of developing breast cancer and ovarian cancer. In fact, about **55-65%** of women with a BRCA1 mutation will develop breast cancer by age 70, compared to the general population risk of about 12%. BRCA1 mutations are also linked to an increased risk of **ovarian cancer**.

- **BRCA2 Mutation**: Similar to BRCA1, a **BRCA2 mutation** also raises the risk of breast cancer, but it is somewhat less aggressive than BRCA1 mutations. Women with a **BRCA2 mutation** have a **45%** risk of developing breast cancer by age 70. Additionally, BRCA2 mutations are associated with other cancers, such as **prostate cancer** in men and **pancreatic cancer**.

Men who inherit a BRCA2 mutation also face an increased risk of developing **breast cancer** (although it's much rarer in men) and **prostate cancer**.

Inherited vs. Sporadic Breast Cancer

While most cases of breast cancer are **sporadic**—meaning they occur by chance and are not inherited—around **5-10%** of breast cancer cases are **familial**, meaning they are linked to inherited genetic mutations.

If someone inherits a mutated BRCA1 or BRCA2 gene, they have a higher risk of developing breast cancer at a younger age and often with more aggressive forms of the disease. It's important to note that **not all breast cancers in families are due to BRCA mutations**, as other genetic factors and environmental influences can contribute to the disease.

Other Genetic Mutations Linked to Breast Cancer

In addition to BRCA1 and BRCA2, there are other inherited genetic mutations that can increase breast cancer risk. Some of the key ones include:

- **TP53 (Li-Fraumeni Syndrome)**: TP53 is a gene that codes for a protein responsible for controlling the cell cycle and preventing damaged cells from multiplying. Mutations in TP53 are associated with a rare inherited condition called **Li-Fraumeni Syndrome**, which increases the risk of various cancers, including breast cancer.

- **PTEN (Cowden Syndrome)**: The PTEN gene helps regulate cell growth and division. Mutations in PTEN lead to a condition called **Cowden Syndrome**, which is linked to an increased risk of breast cancer, as well as other cancers like **endometrial cancer**.

- **PALB2**: This gene works closely with BRCA2 to repair DNA damage. Women with mutations in **PALB2** have an increased risk of breast cancer, sometimes as high as 35-50% by age 70.
- **ATM**: Mutations in the **ATM** gene can increase the risk of breast cancer, particularly in those with a family history of the disease. ATM mutations can lead to problems in repairing DNA damage, similar to BRCA mutations.

Implications of Inherited Mutations

For people with a **family history of breast cancer**, especially if multiple relatives have had the disease at a young age, genetic testing can help determine if there are mutations in genes like BRCA1, BRCA2, or others. Here's why genetic testing is so important:

- **Early Detection**: If you test positive for a **BRCA1 or BRCA2 mutation**, you may be able to take **preventive measures** such as increased surveillance (e.g., more frequent mammograms or MRIs), or even **preventive surgeries** like **mastectomy** (removal of the breasts) or **oophorectomy** (removal of the ovaries) to significantly reduce the risk of developing cancer.

- **Targeted Treatments**: For patients who already have breast cancer and carry BRCA1 or BRCA2 mutations, **targeted therapies** like **PARP inhibitors** can be used. These therapies are designed to block the DNA repair function in cancer cells, which makes them more vulnerable to treatment.

- **Family Screening**: If a mutation is found in a family member, it is important for other family members to undergo genetic counseling and possibly genetic testing as well. Knowing your genetic status can guide decisions about screening and prevention for other relatives.

Genetic Counseling

If you have a family history of breast cancer or have been diagnosed with breast cancer at a young age, **genetic counseling** is recommended. Genetic counselors can help you understand your family's health history, the possible risk of inherited mutations, and the implications of genetic testing. They can also help interpret the results of genetic tests and guide you on the next steps.

You can inherit mutations in the genes that increase your risk of breast cancer, but inheriting a mutation doesn't necessarily mean you will develop the disease. Many factors come into play, including environmental influences, lifestyle choices, and even random mutations. However, knowing whether you carry an inherited mutation can help you make informed decisions about preventive measures and treatment options.

Chapter 3: Prevention and Risk Reduction

Lifestyle Factors

While **genetics** play a major role in determining a person's risk for breast cancer, **lifestyle choices** are just as important. Certain habits can either increase or decrease the likelihood of developing breast cancer. Although we can't change our genetic makeup, we have a significant amount of control over our lifestyle choices, and these choices can influence our overall health, including the risk of breast cancer.

Let's take a look at how **diet, exercise, alcohol consumption,** and **tobacco use** can affect breast cancer risk:

Diet

Eating a balanced and nutritious diet is one of the best ways to improve overall health and reduce the risk of chronic diseases, including cancer. While no single food can prevent or cause breast cancer, certain dietary habits can influence your breast cancer risk:

- **Fatty Diets**: Diets high in **saturated fats**, often found in **red meat, processed foods**, and **full-fat dairy products**, have been linked to an increased risk of breast cancer, particularly in postmenopausal women. This is because high-fat diets can increase **estrogen levels** in the body, which may stimulate the growth of hormone receptor-positive breast cancers.

- **Fruits and Vegetables**: On the flip side, a diet rich in **fruits, vegetables**, and **fiber** can help protect against breast cancer. **Antioxidants**, which are abundant in colorful fruits and vegetables like **berries**, **tomatoes**, and **leafy greens**, help protect cells from damage that could lead to cancer.

- **Phytoestrogens**: Certain plant-based foods, such as **soy**, contain compounds called **phytoestrogens**, which mimic estrogen in the body but are much weaker. While some studies suggest that soy may lower breast cancer risk, particularly in premenopausal women, the research is still mixed. It's best to consume soy foods in moderation as part of a balanced diet.

- **Processed Meat**: **Processed meats** like bacon, sausages, and deli meats have been classified as **carcinogenic** by the World Health Organization (WHO). High consumption of these meats has been linked to an increased risk of several types of cancer, including breast cancer, potentially due to the chemicals used in processing.

- **Alcohol and Sugar**: A diet high in **added sugars** can lead to weight gain and obesity, which are significant risk factors for developing breast cancer. High sugar intake may also contribute to inflammation in the body. Additionally, alcohol consumption can increase the risk of breast cancer, as it affects hormone levels and may directly damage breast tissue.

Exercise

Physical activity is one of the best ways to reduce breast cancer risk, especially for women who are postmenopausal or at higher risk due to family history or genetics.

- **Weight Management**: Regular exercise helps maintain a healthy weight. **Obesity** is a well-known risk factor for breast cancer, particularly after menopause. Fat tissue produces extra estrogen, which can promote the growth of hormone receptor-positive breast cancers. Physical activity helps reduce fat levels and keep estrogen levels in check.

- **Hormonal Benefits**: Exercise can also reduce the amount of circulating estrogen in the body, which may help prevent the development of estrogen-dependent breast cancers. Physical activity, particularly **aerobic exercises** like walking, jogging, or swimming, helps to lower overall hormone levels.

- **Muscle and Bone Health**: In addition to cancer prevention, regular physical activity is great for building and maintaining **strong bones** and **muscles**, reducing the risk of osteoporosis and improving overall health.

- **How Much Exercise?**: The American Cancer Society recommends at least **150 minutes of moderate-intensity exercise** (like brisk walking) or **75 minutes of vigorous-intensity exercise** (like running or cycling) per week. It's also important to include strength training exercises twice a week.

Alcohol Consumption

While **moderate** alcohol consumption may have some cardiovascular benefits, it is also a well-established risk factor for breast cancer. Here's how:

- **How Alcohol Affects the Body**: Alcohol can increase levels of **estrogen** and **other hormones** linked to breast cancer. It may also directly damage DNA, leading to cancerous mutations in breast cells.

- **Increased Risk with Quantity**: The more alcohol a person consumes, the greater their risk. Studies show that **even moderate drinking** (defined as one drink a day for women) can slightly increase breast cancer risk. Drinking more than that—such as two or more drinks daily—raises the risk significantly.

- **The Bottom Line**: Limiting alcohol consumption is a good way to reduce breast cancer risk. The American Cancer Society recommends no more than **one drink per day** for women.

Tobacco Use

Tobacco use is another significant risk factor for many types of cancer, including breast cancer. Smoking is known to damage the DNA in cells, increase inflammation, and contribute to the spread of cancer. Though the connection between smoking and breast cancer is still being studied, several points are clear:

- **Early Smoking and Risk**: Women who **start smoking at a young age** or **smoke heavily** may have a higher risk of developing breast cancer, particularly if they are premenopausal. The toxic chemicals in tobacco can affect breast tissue, leading to mutations that can eventually develop into cancer.

- **Secondhand Smoke**: Women who are **exposed to secondhand smoke** regularly are also at a higher risk of breast cancer, as they may be inhaling the same harmful chemicals that can damage breast tissue.

- **Cigarette Ingredients and Hormones**: Smoking has been shown to **increase estrogen levels**, which is particularly concerning for women with hormone receptor-positive breast cancer. It may also interact with **chemicals in the environment** that can increase the likelihood of cancerous mutations.

- **The Bottom Line**: Quitting smoking is one of the best things you can do for your health and will reduce your risk of breast cancer and many other diseases.

Breastfeeding

Breastfeeding is one of the most natural ways to nourish a baby, but did you know that it can also benefit a mother's health, including reducing her risk of breast cancer? Let's take a closer look at how breastfeeding may reduce the risk of developing breast cancer:

Hormonal Changes During Breastfeeding

When a woman breastfeeds, her body experiences hormonal changes that can help reduce the risk of breast cancer. One of the main factors is the **lower levels of estrogen** during breastfeeding. Estrogen is a hormone that plays a key role in regulating the growth of breast tissue, but **high levels of estrogen** have been linked to an increased risk of hormone receptor-positive breast cancers.

- **Reduced Estrogen Exposure**: While breastfeeding, estrogen levels are naturally lower, which means that the breast tissue does not experience the same rapid growth or cell division that it might during pregnancy without breastfeeding. This decrease in estrogen exposure may reduce the chances of mutations that can lead to cancer.

- **Cell Maturation**: Breastfeeding encourages the **maturation** of breast cells. The longer a woman breastfeeds, the more mature her breast cells become, which may make them less likely to become cancerous. This process involves transforming the cells into a fully differentiated state, which reduces their susceptibility to uncontrolled growth.

Delayed Menstrual Cycles and Reduced Lifetime Exposure to Hormones

Breastfeeding can also affect the frequency of menstrual cycles, which can have an indirect effect on breast cancer risk:

- **Suppressed Ovulation**: During breastfeeding, especially in the first few months, many women experience a delay in the return of their menstrual cycle due to **lactational amenorrhea** (the natural suppression of menstruation). Fewer menstrual cycles mean **less lifetime exposure to estrogen** and other hormones like progesterone. This reduces the cumulative hormonal stimulation of the breast tissue over a woman's lifetime, lowering the risk of developing hormone-related cancers.

- **Longer Interval Between Pregnancies**: Breastfeeding helps delay the return of fertility after childbirth. This can lead to a longer interval between pregnancies, which may also contribute to reduced breast cancer risk. Having multiple pregnancies with extended breastfeeding periods might offer more protection than a woman who has fewer children or shorter breastfeeding durations.

Reduced Risk of Breast Cancer Subtypes

Breastfeeding has been found to reduce the risk of certain types of breast cancer, especially **hormone receptor-positive cancers** (cancers that are fueled by estrogen). This type of cancer is most common in postmenopausal women, but breastfeeding can offer some protection even for women who have had children later in life.

- **Hormone-Receptor-Positive Cancers**: Studies show that breastfeeding may particularly lower the risk of breast cancers that are sensitive to **estrogen** and **progesterone**. These cancers are more likely to be influenced by hormonal changes, which breastfeeding can help modulate.

Longer Duration of Breastfeeding Equals Greater Protection

The more a woman breastfeeds, the greater the potential protective effect against breast cancer. Research suggests that **each year of breastfeeding** can lower a woman's risk of breast cancer by about **4-7%**.

- **Duration Matters**: Women who breastfeed for longer periods—especially for several years across multiple children—tend to have a lower breast cancer risk. Even shorter periods of breastfeeding (several months) have been shown to have some protective effect, though longer durations are more beneficial.

- **Multiple Children**: If a woman has more than one child and breastfeeds them for extended periods, the protection against breast cancer can accumulate. Every additional year of breastfeeding across multiple children can lower the risk further.

Overall Health Benefits of Breastfeeding

Beyond its direct impact on reducing breast cancer risk, breastfeeding offers a host of other health benefits that can support a woman's well-being, indirectly lowering her chances of developing breast cancer:

- **Healthy Weight Management**: Breastfeeding can help new mothers return to their pre-pregnancy weight more quickly. Maintaining a healthy weight is essential for reducing breast cancer risk, as obesity, particularly after menopause, is linked to increased estrogen levels and higher cancer risk.
- **Improved Immune Function**: Breastfeeding boosts a mother's immune system, helping her recover from childbirth and maintaining overall health. This can help protect against various conditions, including cancer.

Hormonal Therapy

Hormonal therapies, including **birth control pills** and **hormone replacement therapy (HRT)**, are widely used to manage reproductive health and the symptoms of menopause. However, their impact on breast cancer risk is a topic of significant concern and ongoing research. Hormones, particularly **estrogen** and **progesterone**, play a central role in the development of some types of breast cancer, which makes understanding their role in hormonal therapies essential for assessing risk.

Birth Control

Birth control pills, or **oral contraceptives**, contain synthetic forms of the hormones estrogen and progesterone (progestin). These hormones are used to prevent pregnancy, regulate menstrual cycles, and manage certain health conditions. However, their use can also influence breast cancer risk.

- **Temporary Increase in Risk**: Research shows that **oral contraceptives** can slightly increase the risk of breast cancer, especially when used in younger women. This increased risk is believed to be linked to the **estrogen and progestin** in the pills, which can stimulate the growth of hormone-sensitive breast tissue.

- **Age of Use**: The risk is higher for women who use birth control at a **younger age**, particularly in their teens and early twenties. The breast tissue during this period is still developing, making it more sensitive to hormonal changes. The longer a woman uses birth control, the greater the exposure to synthetic hormones, and therefore, a slight increase in breast cancer risk may occur.

- **Temporary Nature of Risk**: It's important to note that the increased breast cancer risk linked to birth control is generally temporary. Once a woman stops using hormonal contraception, her risk of breast cancer gradually returns to normal levels within a few years.

- **Other Factors to Consider**: The increased breast cancer risk due to birth control is generally small, especially when compared to other risk factors such as **family history** or **genetic mutations**. Additionally, **non-hormonal contraceptives**, like the IUD (intrauterine device) or barrier methods (condoms), do not carry the same risk for breast cancer.

Women who are at higher risk of breast cancer (due to a family history or genetic mutations like BRCA1/BRCA2) may want to consider **alternative contraception methods**. For most women, the benefits of using birth control (such as preventing pregnancy and regulating periods) typically outweigh the small increase in breast cancer risk.

Hormone Replacement Therapy (HRT)

Hormone replacement therapy (HRT) is commonly used to manage the symptoms of **menopause**, including hot flashes, night sweats, and mood swings. HRT typically combines **estrogen** with **progestin** (for women who still have a uterus) or uses **estrogen-only** therapy for women who have had a hysterectomy.

How HRT affects breast cancer risk:

- **Increased Risk with Combined HRT**: Studies have shown that **combined estrogen and progestin therapy** (the most common form of HRT) **increases the risk of breast cancer**. The risk rises with **long-term use** of HRT, and the increase is more pronounced in women who are over 50 or have been using HRT for several years.

    - **Estrogen's Role**: Estrogen is known to stimulate the growth of certain types of breast cancer, particularly those that are **hormone receptor-positive** (meaning they grow in response to estrogen).

    - **Progestin's Role**: Progestin, a synthetic form of progesterone, is added to protect the uterus from the effects of estrogen. However, it can also contribute to the **promotion of cancerous cell growth** in the breast tissue.

- **Estrogen-Only HRT**: For women who have had a **hysterectomy** and use **estrogen-only HRT**, the

increased breast cancer risk is generally lower than with combined therapy, but it still carries some elevated risk, particularly after several years of use.

- **Breast Cancer Detection and Prognosis**: Some studies have also suggested that women on HRT may experience **later-stage diagnoses** of breast cancer because HRT can mask symptoms or make breast tissue denser, making it harder for mammograms to detect cancer early.

Women considering **HRT** for menopause symptoms should be aware of the risks and discuss them with their doctor, particularly if they have a family history of breast cancer or are at high risk for the disease. For women who need relief from menopausal symptoms, **short-term use** of HRT may be beneficial, but it's essential to limit the duration to minimize the risks. Typically, HRT is recommended for **no longer than 3-5 years**. There are **non-hormonal treatments** available for managing menopausal symptoms, such as antidepressants, **gabapentin** for hot flashes, or lifestyle changes like improving diet and exercise.

Individual Considerations

When it comes to birth control and hormone replacement therapy, **individual risk factors** are crucial in determining whether these treatments are right for a person. Here's a quick overview of considerations:

- **Family History of Breast Cancer**: Women with a family history or genetic mutations such as **BRCA1** or **BRCA2** may have a higher risk of breast cancer. They should discuss alternatives to hormonal therapies with their doctor.

- **Age**: The younger a woman is when she starts hormonal therapies (birth control or HRT), the more significant the risk may be. Women in their **20s or early 30s** who use hormonal contraception may face a slightly higher risk, but the risk generally decreases after stopping.

- **Duration of Use**: The longer a woman uses hormonal contraceptives or HRT, the higher her exposure to hormones. Therefore, **short-term use** is generally safer than prolonged use when it comes to breast cancer risk.

- **Overall Health and Other Risk Factors**: A woman's overall health, weight, lifestyle, and other risk factors (like alcohol use, smoking, or obesity) will also play a role in how hormonal therapies impact breast cancer risk.

Environmental Factors

Exposure to certain chemicals, toxins, and radiation over time can increase the likelihood of developing breast cancer. These environmental influences often interact with your genetic makeup, making some individuals more vulnerable than others.

Environmental Toxins

Many of the chemicals found in everyday products or environmental pollution are linked to cancer, including breast cancer. These chemicals, known as **endocrine disruptors**, interfere with the body's hormone system and can alter normal cell growth and division. The two most common ways they impact breast cancer risk are by mimicking estrogen (a hormone that plays a role in breast tissue development) or blocking the body's natural estrogen receptors.

Common chemicals linked to breast cancer include:

- **BPA (Bisphenol A)**: Found in plastic products, including water bottles and food containers, BPA is one of the most well-known endocrine disruptors. Studies suggest that exposure to BPA can increase the risk of breast cancer by affecting how estrogen works in the body. BPA is often found in food and drink containers, as well as in the lining of some cans.

- **Pesticides and Herbicides**: Pesticides used in agriculture and herbicides sprayed on lawns or around homes contain chemicals such as **DDT (dichlorodiphenyltrichloroethane)**, which is linked to an increased risk of breast cancer. These chemicals persist in the environment and can accumulate in the food chain, leading to prolonged exposure.

- **Phthalates**: These chemicals are used in many products to make plastics more flexible, and they are commonly found in personal care products like shampoos, deodorants, and perfumes. Studies have shown that exposure to phthalates may interfere with hormone production and increase the risk of breast cancer.

- **Polychlorinated Biphenyls (PCBs)**: These industrial chemicals were once widely used in electrical equipment and other products but were banned in many countries in the 1970s due to their harmful environmental impact. Despite the ban, PCBs persist in the environment and have been linked to an increased risk of breast cancer.

- **Toluene and Xylene**: Found in paints, solvents, and cleaning products, these chemicals are toxic when inhaled or absorbed through the skin and have been linked to higher rates of breast cancer. Women who work in environments where these chemicals are used may face a greater risk.

Radiation Exposure

Radiation exposure is another significant environmental factor that can increase the risk of breast cancer. This type of exposure may come from medical treatments, environmental sources, or occupational hazards. Unlike chemical exposure, radiation directly damages DNA in cells, increasing the likelihood of mutations that can lead to cancer:

- **Medical Radiation**: **Chest X-rays**, **CT scans**, and **radiation therapy** used to treat conditions like breast cancer, lymphoma, or other cancers can all increase the risk of developing breast cancer. High-dose radiation, especially during childhood or adolescence, can be particularly harmful to developing breast tissue. Women who have had **radiation therapy** for breast cancer or other cancers may face an increased risk of developing a secondary breast cancer later in life.

- **Environmental Radiation**: Environmental radiation exposure can come from natural sources like **radon**, a colorless, odorless gas found in some homes, particularly those with basements. Radon exposure is the second-leading cause of lung cancer, but research suggests that prolonged exposure can also increase breast cancer risk.

- **Occupational Radiation**: People who work in industries where they are exposed to radiation, such as in nuclear power plants, research facilities, or the medical field, are at a higher risk. Protective measures in the workplace, such as shields and proper equipment, can help reduce this risk.

How Environmental Factors Influence Breast Cancer

The precise mechanisms by which environmental toxins and radiation contribute to breast cancer are still being studied, but several key pathways have been identified.

- **Hormone Disruption:** Many chemicals linked to breast cancer act as **endocrine disruptors**, meaning they mimic or interfere with the body's natural hormones. **Estrogen** is a particularly important hormone in breast cancer risk because it promotes the growth of breast tissue. When the body is exposed to chemicals that mimic estrogen or block its effects, it can lead to abnormal growth of breast cells, increasing the risk of cancer. This is why substances like **BPA, phthalates**, and **PCBs** are often called **xenoestrogens**, or synthetic compounds that mimic the effects of estrogen in the body.

- **DNA Damage:** Radiation, on the other hand, causes **direct DNA damage**. It alters the genetic structure of cells, leading to mutations that can accumulate over time. These mutations can disrupt the normal functioning of cells, leading to **uncontrolled cell growth**, a hallmark of cancer. Unlike other environmental factors that may act slowly over time, radiation exposure can cause immediate and lasting damage to cells, making it one of the most dangerous cancer risk factors.

Reducing Environmental Exposure

While it's impossible to completely eliminate exposure to environmental toxins and radiation, there are several steps you can take to reduce your risk:

Minimize chemical exposure:

- **Choose BPA-free products**: Look for containers labeled as **BPA-free**, especially when purchasing food storage or drink containers. Opt for glass, stainless steel, or other materials that don't contain BPA.

- **Avoid phthalates**: Choose personal care products that are free of phthalates and opt for natural or organic products whenever possible. Check labels for ingredients such as "fragrance" or "parfum," as these often contain phthalates.

- **Eat organic foods**: While the evidence is mixed, some studies suggest that **organic produce** may have lower levels of pesticides, potentially reducing exposure to harmful chemicals. Washing fruits and vegetables thoroughly can also help reduce pesticide residues.

- **Be cautious with cleaning products**: Choose **natural cleaning products** or make your own with ingredients like vinegar and baking soda. Avoid harsh chemical cleaners that contain harmful toxins.

Reduce radiation exposure:

- **Limit unnecessary medical scans**: Only undergo diagnostic imaging like CT scans or X-rays when absolutely necessary. If you need a medical test, ask your doctor about alternatives that expose you to less radiation.

- **Test for radon**: If you live in an area known for radon exposure, consider testing your home with an affordable radon detection kit. If high levels are found, you can install a **radon mitigation system** to reduce the risk.

- **Take precautions in radiation-exposed professions**: If you work in an environment where radiation exposure is a concern, always follow **safety protocols** and wear protective gear, such as lead aprons or gloves, to minimize exposure.

The Importance of Public Health Policies

Governments and organizations play a significant role in reducing environmental risk factors. Public policies such as banning harmful chemicals, regulating industrial emissions, and improving radiation safety standards can help protect entire populations from unnecessary exposure. Ongoing research and advocacy are critical to raising awareness about environmental toxins and pushing for stronger regulations.

Chapter 4: Early Detection and Diagnosis

Screening Methods

Early detection of breast cancer is key to improving treatment outcomes and survival rates. Screening methods help identify potential cancers before symptoms appear. There are several tools and techniques used to detect breast cancer, each with its own strengths and appropriate use cases.

Mammograms

A **mammogram** is an X-ray of the breast tissue and is the most commonly used screening tool for breast cancer. It is highly effective at detecting tumors that are too small to feel and can identify cancers before symptoms occur. During a mammogram, your breasts are compressed between two plates to spread out the tissue, allowing for a clearer image. The compression might be uncomfortable, but it's crucial for obtaining a good image and reducing radiation exposure.

When It's Appropriate

- **Routine Screening**: Mammograms are typically recommended for women over the age of 40, or earlier for those with a family history of breast cancer or other risk factors.
- **Annually or Biennially**: Women with average risk are generally advised to have a mammogram every one or two years, depending on their healthcare provider's recommendation.

- **High-Risk Women**: Women with a strong family history or inherited genetic mutations (like BRCA1 or BRCA2) may begin screening earlier, often starting in their 30s, and may need additional imaging.

Pros and Cons

- **Pros**: Mammograms are quick, widely available, and have been proven to reduce breast cancer mortality by detecting tumors early.
- **Cons**: Mammograms are not perfect. They can sometimes miss small tumors (false negatives), or suggest cancer when there isn't one (false positives). The compression can also be uncomfortable, particularly for women with denser breast tissue.

Ultrasound

An **ultrasound** uses sound waves to create images of the breast tissue. It's often used in conjunction with mammograms to further investigate suspicious areas, particularly in women with dense breasts, where mammograms may be less effective. During an ultrasound, a gel is applied to the skin, and a small device (called a transducer) is moved over the area being examined. The device emits sound waves that bounce off the tissues and create an image. This procedure is non-invasive and painless.

When It's Appropriate

- **Follow-up to a Mammogram**: If a mammogram shows a suspicious area, an ultrasound may be used to determine if the abnormality is a cyst (fluid-filled) or a solid mass (which could be cancerous).

- **Dense Breasts**: For women with dense breast tissue, which can make mammograms less effective, ultrasound may be used to detect tumors that might otherwise be missed.
- **Young Women**: Ultrasound may be used for younger women with denser breasts (typically those under 40), as mammograms can sometimes be less effective due to the higher density of breast tissue in younger women.

Pros and Cons

- **Pros**: Ultrasounds are safe, non-invasive, and can differentiate between solid tumors and benign cysts, reducing unnecessary biopsies.
- **Cons**: Ultrasound does not detect all types of breast cancer, particularly in the early stages. It also does not replace mammography as a primary screening tool.

MRI (Magnetic Resonance Imaging)

An **MRI** is a more advanced imaging technique that uses powerful magnets and radio waves to create detailed images of the breast tissue. MRI is typically used in high-risk women or when a more detailed image is needed to guide treatment decisions. During an MRI, the patient lies face down on a table with the breasts positioned into a special opening. The MRI machine creates a magnetic field and sends radio waves into the body, producing detailed images of the breast tissue. It's typically done after an initial mammogram or ultrasound if there is concern about the presence of cancer.

When It's Appropriate

- **High-Risk Screening**: MRI is recommended for women at high risk of breast cancer, such as those with a family history or known genetic mutations (e.g., BRCA1 or BRCA2).

- **Further Investigation**: When a mammogram or ultrasound raises concerns about a potential cancer, an MRI may be used to gather more information.
- **Evaluating Tumor Size and Spread**: MRI can be useful for assessing the size of the tumor or whether the cancer has spread to other parts of the breast or body.

Pros and Cons

- **Pros**: MRI provides detailed images, making it a powerful tool for detecting cancer, especially in high-risk individuals or those with dense breast tissue. It's highly sensitive and can detect small cancers that may not be visible on a mammogram.
- **Cons**: MRIs are more expensive, less widely available, and may result in false positives, leading to unnecessary biopsies. The procedure also requires the patient to remain still for a long time, which can be uncomfortable.

Biopsy

A **biopsy** is the definitive test for diagnosing breast cancer. It involves removing a small sample of tissue from the breast to be examined under a microscope. A biopsy is usually performed if imaging tests (like mammograms, ultrasound, or MRI) show a suspicious area that needs further investigation.

There are several types of biopsy procedures:

- **Needle Biopsy**: A thin needle is used to remove a small tissue sample. This is the most common method.
- **Core Needle Biopsy**: A larger needle is used to remove a bigger tissue sample, allowing for more accurate results.
- **Surgical Biopsy**: In some cases, a small portion of the lump or area of concern may be removed through surgery.

When It's Appropriate

- **Suspicious Results**: If imaging tests show a lump or abnormal area, a biopsy is done to confirm whether it is cancerous.
- **Determining Cancer Type**: A biopsy helps determine the type of breast cancer, which is crucial for deciding on the appropriate treatment plan.

Pros and Cons

- **Pros**: A biopsy provides a definitive diagnosis, allowing for the determination of whether a tumor is cancerous and what type of cancer it is.
- **Cons**: While generally safe, a biopsy can cause some discomfort, bruising, or bleeding. There is also a small risk of infection.

When to Get Screened

While general guidelines recommend that women begin routine screening in their 40s, it's important to tailor your screening plan to your individual risk factors. Women with a family history of breast cancer, known genetic mutations, or other risk factors should discuss with their healthcare provider when to start screening and which methods are best for them. For those at average risk, mammography is the standard screening tool, but ultrasound or MRI may be considered based on specific circumstances.

Self-Examination

Breast self-examination (BSE) is a simple and important tool that allows you to monitor your own breast health. While it's not a replacement for regular screening methods like mammograms or ultrasounds, doing a monthly self-exam can help you become familiar with the normal look and feel of your breasts, making it easier to notice any changes that might indicate a problem.

What is a Breast Self-Examination?

A breast self-examination involves you checking your own breasts for any changes or abnormalities, such as lumps, changes in size or shape, or skin texture. It's a routine that can be done at home in just a few minutes and helps you stay in tune with your body. The goal is to detect any unusual changes early, which may then be discussed with your healthcare provider.

While most breast lumps aren't cancerous, identifying a new lump or other changes early can help doctors make quicker diagnoses. Early detection of breast cancer can significantly improve the outcome, making self-exams an empowering way to take control of your health.

Here are a few key reasons why breast self-examination matters:

- **Early Detection**: You are the first person who will notice any changes in your body, which means early detection may lead to earlier, more effective treatment.

- **Familiarity with Your Body**: Regular exams help you become familiar with how your breasts normally look and feel. This makes it easier to spot unusual changes.
- **Empowerment**: Taking control of your health and knowing what to look for can provide peace of mind and confidence.

How to Perform a Breast Self-Examination

You can do a breast self-exam in three main steps: looking, feeling, and checking for changes.

Step 1: Look at Your Breasts in the Mirror

- **Position**: Stand in front of a mirror with your shoulders straight and your arms at your sides.
- **What to Look For**:
    - **Shape and Size**: Check for any changes in the size, shape, or symmetry of your breasts. One breast may be slightly larger than the other, but sudden changes or significant differences could be a concern.
    - **Skin Texture**: Look for changes in the skin. Is it dimpled, puckered, or red? These could be signs of underlying issues.
    - **Nipple Changes**: Look for any changes in the nipples, such as inversion (pulling inward), redness, or discharge (other than breast milk if you are nursing).
    - **Visible Lumps or Bulges**: Notice any bulges or lumps in your breast tissue, particularly those that weren't there before.

Step 2: Raise Your Arms and Check Again

- Raise your arms above your head and look for the same signs of change while your arms are in a different position. Sometimes, changes only become noticeable when the breast tissue is stretched out.

Step 3: Feel Your Breasts for Lumps or Abnormalities

- **Position**: Lie down on your back with one arm behind your head. This helps spread the breast tissue evenly across the chest wall.

- **How to Feel**:

  - **Use the pads of your fingers** (not the tips) to gently press down on your breast. Start at the outer edges of your breast and work your way inward in a circular motion.

  - **Move in Patterns**: You can examine your breasts in different patterns—either in concentric circles from the outside in, in a vertical pattern from top to bottom, or in a wedge shape. The important thing is to be thorough and cover all areas of the breast.

  - **Apply Different Pressures**: Use light, medium, and firm pressure as you go along. This will help you feel both the surface and deeper tissues of the breast.

- **What to Look For**:

  - **Lumps or Thickened Areas**: Lumps or hardened tissue could be benign or cancerous, so any new growths should be noted and discussed with your doctor.

- **Tenderness or Pain**: Pay attention to any areas that feel painful, sore, or tender when touched.
- **Unusual Changes in Texture**: Any changes in the texture of the breast tissue, like a hard or lumpy area that doesn't feel like the rest of the tissue, should be checked by a healthcare provider.

Step 4: Check the Area Around the Nipple

- Gently squeeze the nipple to check for any unusual discharge (besides normal breast milk). Discharge that is clear or bloody should be brought to a healthcare professional's attention.

When Should You Perform a Breast Self-Examination?

- **Timing**: Ideally, perform the self-exam once a month, about a week after your period ends, when your breasts are least likely to be swollen or tender.
- **Post-Menopausal Women**: If you're past menopause and no longer have periods, try to do your self-exam on the same day each month to help make it a habit.

What to Do If You Find Something

If you notice a change in your breasts during self-examination, don't panic. Many breast changes are harmless and can be caused by factors like hormonal fluctuations, age, or benign conditions such as cysts or fibroadenomas. However, it's important to see a doctor for further evaluation if:

- You discover a lump or mass.

- Your breasts look or feel different than usual.
- You notice unusual skin changes or nipple discharge.
- Any discomfort or tenderness lasts more than a few weeks.

Your doctor will likely perform a clinical breast exam and may recommend further tests like a mammogram, ultrasound, or biopsy to rule out cancer or other concerns.

Signs and Symptoms

Breast cancer symptoms can vary widely from person to person. While some signs may be obvious and easy to detect, others can be subtle or mistaken for less serious conditions. Being aware of the common—and less common—symptoms of breast cancer is crucial because early detection can lead to better treatment outcomes. Always trust your instincts if something feels off, and consult a healthcare professional if you notice any changes in your breasts.

Common Symptoms of Breast Cancer

1. **Lumps or Masses in the Breast**
    - One of the most well-known signs of breast cancer is the discovery of a lump or mass in the breast. These can feel hard or uneven in texture, and they may not move freely under the skin. However, not all lumps are cancerous. Many benign conditions, like fibrocystic changes or fibroadenomas, can cause lumps as well. If you find a lump that's new or different from the rest of the tissue in your breast, it's important to have it checked by a doctor.

2. **Change in Size or Shape of the Breast**
    - Any noticeable changes in the size or shape of the breast should be taken seriously. For example, if one breast becomes noticeably larger or smaller than the other, or if the skin appears to be pulling inwards, these could be signs of breast cancer. Pay attention to asymmetry that wasn't there before.

3. **Skin Changes**
    - The skin of your breast may undergo changes in texture, color, or appearance. These can include:
        - **Redness** or **swelling**, which could signal inflammation.
        - **Dimpled or puckered skin**, resembling the texture of an orange peel (a condition called **peau d'orange**), which can be a sign of inflammatory breast cancer.
        - **Itchy, scaly skin** or rashes, especially around the nipple, could also signal breast cancer, though they might also be signs of skin conditions like eczema.

4. **Unexplained Pain or Tenderness**
    - Breast pain or tenderness is often linked to hormonal changes, like those during menstruation. However, if the pain doesn't go away after your period or if it's localized to a specific area (especially a new, distinct

pain), it could be a warning sign. It's particularly concerning if the pain is only on one side or if it worsens over time.

5. **Nipple Changes**

    o Any changes in the nipple should be taken seriously, such as:

    - **Nipple inversion** (the nipple turning inward) when it was previously pointing outward.

    - **Nipple discharge** that is clear, bloody, or any discharge that is not breast milk (especially if it's spontaneous or from one breast only).

    - **Redness, soreness, or scaling** around the nipple area (which could resemble an infection but may also indicate **Paget's disease of the breast**, a rare form of breast cancer).

Less Common Symptoms of Breast Cancer

1. **Swelling in the Armpit (Axillary Lymph Nodes)**

    o Swelling or a lump in the armpit could indicate cancer cells spreading to nearby lymph nodes. If you notice any unusual swelling or lumps under your arms that don't go away, it's worth discussing with a doctor.

2. **Persistent Cough or Shortness of Breath**

- Although less common, breast cancer can metastasize (spread) to the lungs, leading to persistent coughing, shortness of breath, or chest pain. These symptoms would most likely be accompanied by other signs, such as weight loss or fatigue.

3. **Unexplained Weight Loss**
    - Sudden or unexplained weight loss—without any changes to diet or exercise—can be a sign of advanced cancer, though it's often associated with other medical conditions.

4. **Fatigue**
    - Extreme tiredness or fatigue that doesn't improve with rest can be a subtle sign of cancer or its treatments. Cancer cells can use up the body's energy, leading to a persistent feeling of exhaustion. It's important to talk to a doctor if you're feeling unusually tired for no apparent reason.

5. **Bone Pain**
    - If breast cancer spreads to the bones, it can cause pain or tenderness in areas like the back, ribs, or hips. This symptom is most common in advanced stages of breast cancer.

6. **Nausea or Loss of Appetite**
    - These symptoms are more often seen in advanced cases of breast cancer, particularly if the cancer has spread to other parts of the body, like the liver. While

nausea and appetite loss can result from many different conditions, it's worth mentioning them to a healthcare provider if they are persistent or unexplained.

When to See a Doctor

If you notice any of the symptoms above—especially if they're new or unusual for you—it's important to see a healthcare provider. While many of these signs can be caused by benign conditions, they should not be ignored. Early detection through a professional evaluation, including a clinical breast exam, imaging tests like mammograms or ultrasounds, or biopsies, is the best way to ensure that any potential issues are addressed as soon as possible. Remember, breast cancer is most treatable when detected early. Keep track of any changes in your body, and don't hesitate to consult a doctor if something doesn't feel right.

The Diagnostic Process

If you've noticed unusual symptoms in your breast or have been referred for a routine screening, understanding the diagnostic process can help reduce the fear of the unknown. While breast cancer can be a daunting diagnosis, advancements in medical imaging and testing allow doctors to detect it early and determine the best treatment options. Here's an summary of the typical steps involved in the breast cancer diagnostic journey, from the first visit to the final diagnosis and staging.

Step 1: Initial Consultation

If you notice any changes in your breast—such as a lump, skin changes, or nipple discharge—it's important to see your healthcare provider as soon as possible. Your doctor will begin by reviewing your medical history, including any risk factors (like family history, personal health history, or lifestyle factors), and asking detailed questions about the symptoms you're experiencing.

During this initial consultation, the doctor will also conduct a **clinical breast exam**, in which they'll physically examine your breasts, underarms, and collarbone for signs of lumps, swelling, or other abnormalities. This step helps the doctor determine whether further testing is needed.

Step 2: Imaging Tests

If a physical exam raises concerns, the next step in the diagnostic process is usually imaging. The goal is to get a clearer view of the breast tissue to determine if there are any signs of cancer or other conditions. Here are the most common imaging tests used to diagnose breast cancer:

1. Mammogram

- **What It Is**: A mammogram is an X-ray of the breast. It's one of the most common and effective ways to screen for breast cancer.

- **Why It's Done**: Mammograms can detect abnormal growths in the breast, even before they can be felt. Regular screening is recommended for women over 40, or earlier if they have higher risk factors.

- **What It Shows**: It can identify masses, calcifications (small clusters of calcium), or other signs that might suggest cancer.

- **How It's Done**: During a mammogram, the breast is placed between two plates, which compress the breast to get clear X-ray images. The process can be slightly uncomfortable but usually takes only a few minutes.

2. Ultrasound

- **What It Is**: An ultrasound uses sound waves to create images of the breast tissue. It's often used in combination with mammography.

- **Why It's Done**: If a mammogram finds an abnormality, an ultrasound can help determine whether the abnormality is a solid mass (which could be cancerous) or a fluid-filled cyst (which is usually benign).

- **What It Shows**: It provides a clear image of the size, shape, and boundaries of any lumps or masses and can help guide biopsies.

- **How It's Done**: A gel is applied to the breast, and a small device called a transducer is moved over the area to capture images.

3. Magnetic Resonance Imaging (MRI)

- **What It Is**: MRI uses powerful magnets and radio waves to produce detailed images of the breast tissue. It's particularly useful in women with dense breast tissue or those at high risk for breast cancer.

- **Why It's Done**: An MRI is usually used to get more detailed images after a mammogram or ultrasound, or when there's concern about how far cancer has spread.

- **What It Shows**: It helps doctors assess the size of a tumor, its location, and if cancer has spread to other tissues.

- **How It's Done**: You'll lie down on a table, and a contrast dye is injected into your veins. You will then enter the MRI machine, which takes detailed images while you remain still for several minutes.

Step 3: Biopsy

If imaging tests suggest a possible tumor or abnormality, the next step is typically a **biopsy**, where a sample of the suspicious tissue is taken and examined under a microscope. A biopsy is the only way to confirm whether cancer is present.

What It Is

- A biopsy involves removing a small piece of tissue from the breast for laboratory testing. The sample will be analyzed to determine whether cancer cells are present and, if so, what type of cancer it is.

Types of Biopsy

1. **Fine Needle Aspiration (FNA)**: A thin, hollow needle is used to remove a small amount of tissue or fluid from the suspicious area.
2. **Core Needle Biopsy**: A larger needle is used to remove a bigger tissue sample from the lump or abnormal area.
3. **Surgical Biopsy**: If the other methods are inconclusive, a small surgical incision is made to remove the entire lump or a portion of it.

The biopsy will help determine whether the abnormal growth is cancerous, as well as provide important information about the cancer type and its characteristics (such as whether it is hormone receptor-positive or HER2-positive).

Step 4: Staging the Cancer

Once a biopsy confirms cancer, doctors will move on to **staging** the cancer. Staging tells doctors how far the cancer has spread and helps them develop the best treatment plan.

The **staging process** typically includes imaging tests to look for cancer in other parts of the body, such as the lymph nodes, bones, liver, or lungs. These can include:

- **CT scans**: To look for cancer spread to the lungs, liver, or other organs.
- **Bone scans**: To check for cancer spread to the bones.
- **PET scans**: To detect any active cancer cells in the body.
- **Sentinel lymph node biopsy**: This test determines whether cancer has spread to the lymph nodes nearest to the tumor in the breast.

The stages of breast cancer are generally broken down as follows:

- **Stage 0**: Non-invasive (in situ) cancer, like ductal carcinoma in situ (DCIS), where the cancer cells haven't spread outside the ducts or lobules.
- **Stage I**: Early stage where the tumor is small (up to 2 cm) and has not spread to the lymph nodes.
- **Stage II**: The tumor may be larger or have spread to a few nearby lymph nodes.
- **Stage III**: Larger tumors or extensive lymph node involvement, with possible spread to nearby tissues.
- **Stage IV**: Metastatic breast cancer, where the cancer has spread to other parts of the body, such as the lungs, liver, or bones.

Step 5: Final Diagnosis and Treatment Plan

After the staging process, doctors can assess the cancer's exact characteristics, including the **molecular subtype** (such as hormone receptor-positive, HER2-positive, or triple-negative), and create a treatment plan based on the specific type of cancer.

Treatment plans often include a combination of surgery, radiation therapy, chemotherapy, hormone therapy, or targeted therapy, depending on the stage and subtype of breast cancer. Your doctor will explain the treatment options available to you and discuss the best course of action.

Chapter 5: Staging and Prognosis

Understanding Breast Cancer Staging

Staging is a crucial part of breast cancer diagnosis. It describes the extent to which the cancer has spread, helping doctors determine how advanced the disease is and what treatments will be most effective. The stage of the cancer is determined based on several factors, including the size of the tumor, whether the cancer has spread to nearby lymph nodes, and if it has spread to other parts of the body. Staging not only guides treatment decisions but also plays a significant role in predicting the patient's prognosis.

Breast cancer is staged from **Stage 0** (non-invasive) to **Stage IV** (advanced, metastatic cancer). Here's a breakdown of each stage and what it means for prognosis.

Stage 0: Carcinoma In Situ

What It Is:

- **Stage 0** is the earliest form of breast cancer, often referred to as **non-invasive** or **in situ** cancer.

- This stage includes conditions like **ductal carcinoma in situ (DCIS)** and **lobular carcinoma in situ (LCIS)**, where abnormal cells are found but have not spread beyond the ducts or lobules where they originated.

Prognosis:

- The prognosis for Stage 0 breast cancer is **excellent**. Since the cancer is localized and hasn't spread, it is highly treatable, and the survival rate is very high.

- The goal at this stage is often to remove the abnormal cells and monitor the area for any signs of recurrence.

Treatment:

- Treatment often involves surgery to remove the abnormal tissue, and sometimes radiation or hormone therapy, depending on the individual case.

Stage I: Early-Stage Invasive Cancer

What It Is:

- **Stage I** breast cancer is considered early-stage and **invasive**, meaning the cancer cells have started to spread beyond the ducts or lobules into surrounding breast tissue.
- At this stage, the tumor is **small** (up to 2 cm) and has not spread to lymph nodes or other parts of the body.

Prognosis:

- The prognosis for Stage I breast cancer is **very good**, with a high survival rate due to early detection and treatment.
- The 5-year survival rate for Stage I breast cancer is over **90%**. Most people at this stage can expect a favorable outcome.

Treatment:

- Surgery to remove the tumor (either a lumpectomy or mastectomy) is typically the primary treatment. Radiation therapy is often recommended afterward to reduce the risk of recurrence.

- Depending on the cancer's molecular subtype (e.g., hormone receptor-positive, HER2-positive), hormone therapy or targeted therapy may also be recommended.

Stage II: Locally Advanced Cancer

What It Is:

- **Stage II** is a locally advanced form of breast cancer, where the tumor is **larger** (between 2 and 5 cm) or has spread to **a few nearby lymph nodes** but not to distant areas of the body.
- This stage can also include tumors smaller than 2 cm if there is significant spread to the lymph nodes.

Prognosis:

- The prognosis for Stage II breast cancer is still relatively good, with a 5-year survival rate between **70% to 90%**, depending on factors like tumor size, lymph node involvement, and cancer subtype.
- Treatment is more aggressive than Stage I due to the involvement of lymph nodes, but survival rates remain high when treatment is started early.

Treatment:

- Treatment often involves a combination of surgery, chemotherapy, radiation, and sometimes hormone therapy or targeted therapy.
- Neoadjuvant therapy (chemotherapy before surgery) may be recommended to shrink the tumor before removal.

Stage III: Advanced Localized Cancer

What It Is:

- **Stage III** is a more advanced form of locally invasive breast cancer, where the tumor is **large** (larger than 5 cm) or has spread extensively to nearby lymph nodes, chest wall, or skin.
- This stage does not involve distant metastasis (spread to other parts of the body), but the cancer is more extensive in the breast and surrounding areas.

Prognosis:

- The prognosis for Stage III breast cancer is less favorable than Stage I or II, but still treatable. The 5-year survival rate for Stage III is around **50% to 70%**.
- Treatment is more intensive at this stage, and while the cancer is still confined to the breast area, it requires a combination of therapies to prevent recurrence or spread.

Treatment:

- Stage III cancer is often treated with chemotherapy (usually both before and after surgery), surgery to remove the tumor, and radiation therapy.
- Hormone therapy or HER2-targeted therapies may also be used, depending on the cancer's molecular subtype.

Stage IV: Metastatic Cancer

What It Is:

- **Stage IV** breast cancer is **metastatic**, meaning the cancer has spread to other parts of the body, such as the lungs, liver, bones, or brain.
- The cancer may have initially started in the breast but has now spread to distant organs or tissues.

Prognosis:

- The prognosis for Stage IV breast cancer is more guarded. The 5-year survival rate for Stage IV is significantly lower than earlier stages, typically around **20% to 30%**.
- While Stage IV breast cancer is not considered curable, treatment can help control the disease and improve quality of life for many people.

Treatment:

- At Stage IV, treatment focuses on controlling the cancer and improving symptoms. Treatment may include chemotherapy, targeted therapy, hormone therapy, immunotherapy, and sometimes surgery to relieve symptoms.
- Treatment may not completely eliminate the cancer but aims to slow its growth and spread, extend life, and manage pain or other side effects.

Factors Affecting Prognosis

While staging is the most important factor in determining prognosis, several other aspects can affect how well a person responds to treatment, including:

1. **Molecular Subtype**: Tumors that are hormone receptor-positive or HER2-positive tend to respond better to specific treatments like hormone therapy or targeted therapies.
2. **Age**: Younger patients tend to have a more aggressive form of breast cancer, but they may also respond better to treatment.
3. **Overall Health**: A person's general health can influence how well they tolerate treatments and their likelihood of recovery.
4. **Response to Treatment**: The way a tumor responds to initial treatment can indicate how well it might respond to ongoing therapies.

Lymph Node Involvement

Lymph nodes play a critical role in the staging and prognosis of breast cancer. These small, bean-shaped structures are part of the **lymphatic system**, which is a network of tissues and organs that help the body fight infection and disease. Lymph nodes act as filters, trapping harmful substances like bacteria, viruses, and cancer cells, and are often the first place cancer cells spread when they leave the original tumor.

In breast cancer, the **presence or absence of cancer in the lymph nodes** is a key factor that helps determine the stage of the disease and guides treatment decisions. Here's a breakdown of the significance of lymph node involvement:

What Are Lymph Nodes, and Why Do They Matter?

- Lymph nodes are located throughout the body, including under the arms (axillary lymph nodes), around the collarbone (supraclavicular nodes), and near the breastbone (internal mammary nodes).

- The **axillary lymph nodes** are the most commonly involved in breast cancer because they are located close to the breast tissue and serve as the first line of defense against cancerous cells that break away from the tumor.
- If cancer cells break away from the primary tumor in the breast, they may travel through the lymphatic system and settle in nearby lymph nodes. The more lymph nodes affected, the more likely it is that the cancer could spread to other parts of the body.

How Lymph Node Involvement Affects Breast Cancer Staging

Lymph node involvement is a critical part of **breast cancer staging**. The presence of cancer in the lymph nodes helps determine the stage of the disease, which ranges from **Stage 0** (non-invasive) to **Stage IV** (metastatic). Here's how it works:

- **No Lymph Node Involvement (N0):** If the cancer has not spread to any lymph nodes, it is staged as **N0**. This is generally a sign of early-stage breast cancer and usually results in a **better prognosis** because it indicates the cancer has not spread to other parts of the body.
- **Lymph Node Involvement (N1, N2, N3):** If cancer cells are found in nearby lymph nodes, it is staged as **N1**, **N2**, or **N3**, with the number of affected nodes influencing the stage. The more lymph nodes involved, the higher the stage and the more aggressive the treatment plan may need to be.

The Impact of Lymph Node Involvement on Prognosis

Lymph node involvement has a significant impact on the **prognosis** of breast cancer, as it indicates whether the cancer has started to spread beyond the primary tumor site. The more lymph nodes affected, the more likely the cancer has spread to other parts of the body, which can make treatment more challenging.

Here's how lymph node involvement influences prognosis:

1. **Fewer Affected Lymph Nodes (1-3):**

    o If cancer is found in only **1 to 3 lymph nodes**, the prognosis is generally **favorable**. The cancer is still considered **locally advanced**, but it may be treatable with surgery, chemotherapy, and possibly radiation.

    o The 5-year survival rate is typically **high** in this group, especially if the cancer is hormone receptor-positive or HER2-positive, as these subtypes respond well to targeted treatments.

2. **More Affected Lymph Nodes (4 or More):**

    o If **4 or more lymph nodes** are involved, the cancer is considered to have spread more extensively. This often suggests a more **aggressive disease**, and the prognosis may be **less favorable**.

    o In these cases, treatment may include a combination of surgery, chemotherapy, radiation, and sometimes immunotherapy or targeted therapies. The survival rate may be lower than for people with fewer lymph nodes affected, but survival rates have improved with advances in treatment.

3. **Involvement of Distant Lymph Nodes:**

    o If cancer spreads to **distant lymph nodes**, such as those near the collarbone or under the breastbone, the disease may be classified as **Stage III or Stage IV**, meaning the cancer is more advanced and metastatic.

    o This type of involvement often requires a more intensive treatment plan and may impact prognosis more significantly.

How Lymph Node Involvement Influences Treatment

The extent of lymph node involvement not only affects prognosis but also **guides treatment decisions**. Here's how it works:

- **Surgical Options:** If cancer is found in nearby lymph nodes, surgery may be required to remove them, along with the primary tumor. This procedure, called a **lymph node dissection**, helps prevent further spread of cancer and can improve outcomes.

- **Radiation Therapy:** When cancer is found in the lymph nodes, doctors may recommend **radiation therapy** to the area of the lymph nodes, even after surgery, to destroy any remaining cancer cells and reduce the risk of recurrence.

- **Chemotherapy and Targeted Therapies:** If the cancer has spread to lymph nodes, **chemotherapy** may be recommended to target cancer cells throughout the body. In some cases, **targeted therapies** (such as HER2-targeted treatments) may also be used to treat specific types of cancer based on the molecular characteristics of the tumor.

- **Hormone Therapy:** If the cancer is **hormone receptor-positive** (meaning it depends on hormones like estrogen or progesterone to grow), hormone therapy can be used to block these hormones and reduce the risk of the cancer coming back.

Prognostic Factors

When a person is diagnosed with breast cancer, doctors assess several factors to predict the likely course of the disease and the chance of recovery. These factors, called **prognostic factors**, help doctors develop a personalized treatment plan and provide an estimate of the patient's overall outlook. Here, we'll take a closer look at some of the most important prognostic factors, including tumor grade, receptor status, and overall health.

Tumor Grade: How Aggressive Is the Cancer?

The **tumor grade** refers to how abnormal the cancer cells look under a microscope and how quickly the tumor is likely to grow. A tumor's grade can provide an idea of how aggressive or slow-growing the cancer is.

- **Grade 1 (Low grade):** The cancer cells look more like normal cells and tend to grow slowly. This is often a sign of a **less aggressive** tumor and usually results in a better prognosis.

- **Grade 2 (Intermediate grade):** The cancer cells look somewhat abnormal and tend to grow at a moderate rate. This is considered an **intermediate risk** for the cancer's spread.

- **Grade 3 (High grade):** The cancer cells look very abnormal and tend to grow rapidly. High-grade tumors are typically **more aggressive** and may spread more quickly, which can lead to a **poorer prognosis**.

Tumor grade is an important factor that helps doctors predict how the cancer might behave, which impacts treatment decisions. Generally, low-grade tumors have a better outlook, while high-grade tumors require more intensive treatments.

Receptor Status: Does the Tumor Respond to Hormones or Targeted Treatments?

Breast cancer cells have receptors on their surface that can influence how the cancer behaves and how well it responds to certain treatments. The two most important receptor types in breast cancer are **estrogen receptors (ER)** and **HER2 receptors**.

- **Estrogen Receptor-Positive (ER+):** In many breast cancers, the cancer cells have **estrogen receptors** that allow the hormone estrogen to fuel the growth of the tumor. If the tumor is ER-positive, it is often treated with **hormone therapy** (like tamoxifen or aromatase inhibitors) that blocks estrogen's effects. ER-positive breast cancer typically has a better prognosis because it's often less aggressive and more treatable.

- **Progesterone Receptor-Positive (PR+):** Some breast cancers are **progesterone receptor-positive** as well. Like ER-positive tumors, PR-positive tumors tend to grow more slowly and respond well to hormone therapy.

- **HER2-Positive:** HER2 is a protein that promotes cancer cell growth. In about **20% of breast cancers**, the tumor cells produce too much HER2, making the cancer grow and spread more quickly. However, HER2-positive cancers can be treated with targeted therapies (like trastuzumab or Herceptin) that block HER2 and slow the cancer's growth. Despite being more aggressive, HER2-positive breast cancer can often be treated successfully with the right medications, which improves the prognosis.

- **Triple-Negative Breast Cancer (TNBC):** This type of breast cancer lacks all three of these receptors (ER, PR, and HER2). As a result, it doesn't respond to hormone therapies or HER2-targeted treatments, making it more challenging to treat. However, **chemotherapy** and sometimes **immunotherapy** are used to treat TNBC, and outcomes can vary widely depending on how aggressive the cancer is and the overall health of the patient.

The **receptor status** is one of the most crucial factors in determining the type of treatment a patient will receive and the likely outcome of their disease. Tumors that are ER-positive, PR-positive, or HER2-positive often have a better prognosis because they are more likely to respond to targeted therapies.

Tumor Size: How Large Is the Tumor?

The size of the tumor at diagnosis also plays a critical role in determining prognosis. In general, the **larger the tumor**, the more likely it has spread to nearby tissues or lymph nodes, which can affect the outcome. Here's what you need to know:

- **Smaller Tumors (Stage 1):** Tumors that are small (less than 2 cm) and confined to the breast tend to have a better prognosis because they are less likely to have spread to lymph nodes or distant organs.
- **Larger Tumors (Stage 2 and above):** Larger tumors (greater than 2 cm) are more likely to have invaded surrounding tissues and possibly spread to the lymph nodes. This increases the risk of recurrence and can make treatment more complex.

Smaller tumors are typically associated with better outcomes and a lower risk of recurrence, especially if caught early.

Lymph Node Involvement: Has the Cancer Spread to Lymph Nodes?

As discussed earlier, **lymph nodes** are often the first place breast cancer spreads. If cancer cells have spread to nearby lymph nodes, this is an important factor in assessing the prognosis:

- **No Lymph Node Involvement (N0):** If cancer hasn't spread to the lymph nodes, the prognosis is generally better, and the chance of recurrence is lower.
- **Lymph Node Involvement (N1, N2, N3):** The more lymph nodes that are affected, the higher the stage of the cancer, and the greater the chance of recurrence. Lymph node involvement often indicates that the cancer has spread beyond the breast and requires more aggressive treatment.

Lymph node involvement is a critical part of staging and directly impacts the **treatment approach** and **prognosis**.

Overall Health: What is the Patient's Health Like?

A person's overall health can influence their ability to tolerate treatment and their chances of recovery. Here are some factors related to overall health:

- **Age:** Younger women generally have a better prognosis because their bodies are often more responsive to treatment and recovery. However, breast cancer in younger women (especially under 40) is often more aggressive and harder to treat. In older women, the cancer may be less aggressive, but other health conditions may complicate treatment.

- **Co-existing Health Conditions:** If a person has other health conditions, like heart disease, diabetes, or obesity, it may impact their ability to undergo certain treatments, such as chemotherapy. This can affect overall treatment success and prognosis.

- **Fitness Level:** Women who are physically fit and maintain a healthy lifestyle are often better able to tolerate the side effects of cancer treatments and may recover more quickly.

Overall health factors, such as the presence of other diseases or physical condition, can impact how the body responds to treatment and its ability to fight cancer, which in turn can influence **prognosis**.

Other Factors:

There are additional factors that can influence breast cancer outcomes:

- **Age at Diagnosis:** Younger women tend to have more aggressive forms of breast cancer, but they also tend to tolerate treatments better. Older women may have slower-growing cancers but could be more vulnerable to complications during treatment.

- **Hormone Therapy Response:** Whether the cancer responds to hormone therapy or targeted treatments like HER2 inhibitors can also affect prognosis. Hormone receptor-positive cancers often have a better long-term outlook.

The Role of Molecular Testing

In recent years, advancements in **molecular testing** have revolutionized the way doctors understand and treat breast cancer. These tests help identify the **genetic and molecular makeup** of the cancer, offering a deeper insight into its behavior, aggressiveness, and how it might respond to different treatments. While traditional methods like biopsies and imaging focus on the physical aspects of the tumor, **molecular testing** digs deeper into the **cellular level**, allowing for a more **personalized approach** to care.

What is Molecular Testing?

Molecular testing refers to a variety of tests that look at the **genes**, **proteins**, and other molecules within the cancer cells to determine specific characteristics that can influence how the cancer behaves. By analyzing these molecular markers, doctors can better understand the cancer's **genetic profile**, predict how it might grow or spread, and select the most effective treatment options.

These tests can be done on tumor samples taken during a **biopsy** or surgery, or even from a **blood sample** in some cases. The results from molecular testing can provide essential information on how to **tailor treatment** to an individual's cancer, which is sometimes referred to as **precision medicine**.

How Does Molecular Testing Help?

Molecular testing can play a pivotal role in predicting how aggressive the cancer is, whether it will respond to certain therapies, and what the prognosis might be. Let's explore some of the key areas where molecular testing can make a difference:

1. Predicting Cancer Behavior

Molecular tests can help predict how fast a cancer is likely to grow and whether it has the potential to spread (metastasize). By identifying certain genetic mutations or markers, doctors can assess if the cancer is more likely to behave aggressively or if it will grow more slowly. This can help patients and doctors make informed decisions about the best course of action—whether the cancer requires more aggressive treatment or if a less invasive approach is appropriate.

2. Identifying Targeted Therapies

One of the most exciting aspects of molecular testing is its ability to identify specific mutations or molecular markers in cancer cells that can be targeted with **precision treatments**. For example:

- **HER2 Testing:** About 20% of breast cancers have too much of a protein called HER2, which drives the cancer's growth. If a tumor tests positive for HER2, drugs like **trastuzumab** (Herceptin) can be used to block HER2 receptors, slowing the cancer's growth.

- **Hormone Receptor Testing:** In breast cancers that are **estrogen receptor-positive (ER+)** or **progesterone receptor-positive (PR+)**, hormone-blocking therapies like **tamoxifen** or **aromatase inhibitors** can stop the cancer cells from growing by blocking these hormones.

Molecular testing helps ensure that patients receive the treatments most likely to work for their specific cancer.

3. Assessing the Likelihood of Recurrence

Molecular testing can also be used to evaluate the risk of cancer returning after treatment. Some molecular tests measure the **gene expression** of the tumor, revealing patterns that indicate whether the cancer is likely to come back in the future. Tests like **Oncotype DX** and **MammaPrint** analyze a tumor's genetic profile and assign a recurrence score, helping doctors decide whether a patient may benefit from additional treatments, such as chemotherapy, or if less aggressive treatment will suffice.

4. Personalizing Treatment Plans

Every patient is unique, and so is every cancer. Molecular testing provides information that helps doctors create **personalized treatment plans** based on the specific characteristics of the patient's cancer. For example, if a tumor tests positive for a certain genetic mutation or protein, doctors may choose to treat the cancer with a **targeted therapy** that is known to work well with that specific genetic alteration.

This tailored approach not only increases the chances of success but also minimizes unnecessary treatments that may be less effective, leading to fewer side effects and a better overall quality of life for the patient.

Common Types of Molecular Tests for Breast Cancer

There are several different molecular tests available, each serving a unique purpose in the diagnosis and treatment of breast cancer. Some of the most common include:

1. HER2 Testing

As mentioned earlier, **HER2-positive** cancers have an overproduction of the HER2 protein, which makes the cancer cells grow uncontrollably. HER2 testing is done to determine whether this protein is present in large quantities, which can guide treatment decisions, particularly the use of **targeted therapies** such as Herceptin.

2. Hormone Receptor Testing (ER/PR)

This test checks for the presence of estrogen (ER) and progesterone (PR) receptors on cancer cells. Cancers that are **ER+ or PR+** can be treated with hormone therapy, which blocks the hormones from fueling cancer growth.

3. Genetic Testing for Mutations (e.g., BRCA1, BRCA2)

Some genetic mutations, particularly **BRCA1** and **BRCA2**, increase the risk of breast cancer. If a patient tests positive for these mutations, it may change the way doctors approach treatment. For example, women with BRCA mutations might be offered more aggressive treatments or even preventive measures (like surgery or medication) to reduce the risk of cancer recurrence.

4. Genomic Tests (e.g., Oncotype DX, MammaPrint)

Genomic tests look at the activity of specific genes in the tumor to assess the likelihood of recurrence and predict how the tumor might respond to different treatments. These tests can help identify patients who may not need chemotherapy after surgery, based on the tumor's genetic profile.

5. Next-Generation Sequencing (NGS)

Next-Generation Sequencing is an advanced molecular test that looks for mutations in a wide range of genes, providing a comprehensive look at a patient's tumor. This test can detect both common and rare genetic alterations, and it is increasingly being used to identify treatment options for patients with **metastatic breast cancer** or cancers that are resistant to traditional therapies.

Why Molecular Testing Matters

Molecular testing is critical because it allows for a **tailored approach** to breast cancer treatment, ensuring that patients receive the most effective therapies while avoiding unnecessary treatments. It can help:

- Predict how the cancer will behave
- Identify the most effective treatments
- Guide decisions about the need for chemotherapy, hormone therapy, or targeted therapies
- Help detect early signs of recurrence

By understanding the unique genetic and molecular characteristics of breast cancer, doctors can offer more **precise and personalized treatment**, improving the chance of successful outcomes and reducing the risk of side effects.

Chapter 6: Treatment Options

Surgery

When it comes to treating breast cancer, surgery is often a critical part of the treatment plan. The goal of surgery is to remove the tumor or the entire breast (depending on the case), with the aim of eliminating cancer cells and preventing the cancer from spreading. There are different types of surgical options available, each with its own set of benefits and considerations.

Lumpectomy

A **lumpectomy**, also known as **breast-conserving surgery**, involves removing the cancerous tumor along with a small margin of healthy tissue around it. This procedure aims to preserve as much of the breast as possible, making it an appealing option for many women who want to retain their breast shape.

What Does the Procedure Involve?

During a lumpectomy, only the tumor and a surrounding area of healthy tissue are removed. The size of the tumor and its location in the breast will determine the extent of the surgery. In some cases, several lymph nodes near the tumor may also be removed to check for cancer spread (this is called **sentinel lymph node biopsy**).

After the tumor is removed, a pathologist examines the tissue to ensure that all cancer cells have been taken out. In some instances, the surgery may be followed by additional treatments such as **radiation therapy** to destroy any remaining cancer cells in the breast.

Benefits of Lumpectomy:

- **Preserves the breast:** Most women are able to keep their breast and its appearance, though there may be some cosmetic changes.
- **Faster recovery:** Compared to a mastectomy, a lumpectomy typically requires a shorter hospital stay and a quicker recovery time.
- **Less invasive:** It is a less invasive surgery compared to a mastectomy, which may be important for some women in terms of maintaining their sense of body image.

Considerations:

- After a lumpectomy, most women will need **radiation therapy** to ensure that any remaining cancer cells are destroyed. Radiation is often recommended after breast-conserving surgery to reduce the risk of the cancer returning in the same breast.
- In some cases, if the tumor is large relative to the size of the breast or if there are multiple tumors, a lumpectomy may not be possible or effective.

Mastectomy: Removing the Entire Breast

A **mastectomy** involves the removal of the entire breast, including the nipple, areola, and most of the breast tissue. This procedure is often recommended if the cancer is widespread or if there are multiple areas of cancer within the breast. It may also be considered if a woman has a high risk of cancer recurrence or if she has a genetic mutation (like **BRCA1** or **BRCA2**) that increases her risk of developing breast cancer in both breasts.

What Does the Procedure Involve?

During a mastectomy, the entire breast tissue is removed. In some cases, nearby lymph nodes or chest muscles may also be removed, depending on the spread of the cancer. There are different types of mastectomies, including:

- **Total (simple) mastectomy:** Removes the entire breast tissue but does not involve the removal of lymph nodes or muscles.

- **Modified radical mastectomy:** Removes the entire breast along with some of the lymph nodes under the arm. The chest muscles are usually left intact.

- **Radical mastectomy:** A more extensive surgery where the entire breast, lymph nodes, and chest muscles are removed. This is now rarely done and is typically reserved for more advanced cancers.

Benefits of Mastectomy:

- **Completely removes the breast tissue:** A mastectomy may offer peace of mind to women whose cancer is more widespread or who have a higher risk of recurrence.

- **Lower recurrence rates:** For women with larger or more aggressive tumors, a mastectomy can lower the risk of cancer coming back in the same breast.

Considerations:

- **Physical and emotional impact:** While a mastectomy is highly effective in removing the cancer, it can be an emotionally challenging experience for many women due to the loss of a breast. However, **breast reconstruction** options are available to help restore breast appearance.

- **Longer recovery time:** Mastectomy surgery generally requires a longer recovery time than lumpectomy, and it can also be more physically demanding.
- **Possible side effects:** Some women may experience complications like **seroma** (fluid buildup), **infection**, or changes in arm function if lymph nodes are removed.

Breast Reconstruction: Restoring Appearance After Surgery

For many women, breast reconstruction is an essential part of their recovery after a mastectomy. This procedure helps rebuild the breast to restore its shape and appearance, improving body image and emotional well-being.

What Does Breast Reconstruction Involve?

Breast reconstruction can be done immediately after the mastectomy or at a later date, depending on the patient's preferences and health status. The two primary types of reconstruction are:

- **Implant-based reconstruction:** Involves placing silicone or saline implants under the skin or chest muscle to recreate the shape of the breast. This is the most common type of breast reconstruction.
- **Autologous (flap) reconstruction:** Involves using tissue from another part of the body (like the abdomen, back, or thighs) to rebuild the breast. This type of reconstruction can offer more natural results and is an option for women who may not be candidates for implants.

Benefits of Breast Reconstruction:

- **Restores breast shape:** For women who want to regain their body image after a mastectomy, breast reconstruction can help restore the look of the breast.
- **Improves emotional well-being:** Many women report feeling more confident and positive about their appearance after reconstruction, which can be an important part of their emotional healing.
- **Immediate or delayed options:** Reconstruction can be done either immediately after mastectomy or later, depending on individual preferences and circumstances.

Considerations:

- **Complexity of surgery:** Breast reconstruction is a complex procedure that may involve multiple surgeries over several months or years. Recovery can take time, and there may be a risk of complications such as infection or issues with the implants or tissue.
- **Not all women opt for reconstruction:** Some women choose not to undergo breast reconstruction for personal or medical reasons, and this decision is entirely their own. Prostheses (artificial breasts) can also be used as an alternative.

Making the Right Choice: What to Consider

Choosing the right surgical option is a deeply personal decision that depends on various factors, including the stage and type of cancer, the patient's overall health, body image preferences, and emotional needs. It's important to discuss the options with a healthcare team, including a **breast**

surgeon, **oncologist**, and **plastic surgeon**, who can provide guidance and help weigh the pros and cons of each option.

- **Lumpectomy** is a good option for early-stage cancers and those who want to preserve the appearance of the breast.
- **Mastectomy** may be recommended for larger or more aggressive cancers, or for women with a high risk of recurrence.
- **Breast reconstruction** can help restore a woman's physical appearance and emotional well-being after a mastectomy.

Ultimately, the decision about surgery should be based on the patient's unique circumstances, and it's important to consider both the physical and emotional aspects of each option.

Radiation Therapy

Radiation therapy is a powerful treatment option used to destroy cancer cells and shrink tumors by using high-energy rays, similar to X-rays. For breast cancer, it plays a crucial role in both treating the cancer directly and preventing it from returning.

What Is Radiation Therapy?

Radiation therapy, often just called **radiotherapy**, uses targeted beams of radiation to kill or damage cancer cells. The goal is to destroy the cancer cells in the breast or surrounding areas while minimizing damage to healthy tissue. It's a localized treatment, meaning it targets only the area that needs it, and the effects are limited to that region.

There are two main types of radiation therapy used for breast cancer:

1. **External Beam Radiation Therapy** (EBRT): This is the most common form used for breast cancer. The radiation is delivered from a machine outside the body, which directs the radiation beams to the tumor site. It's a non-invasive treatment that requires no incisions.

2. **Brachytherapy** (Internal Radiation): This type of radiation therapy involves placing radioactive material directly inside or near the tumor. It's used in specific cases, like for women who've had a lumpectomy for early-stage breast cancer.

When Is Radiation Therapy Needed?

Radiation therapy is commonly used in the following situations:

1. **After Surgery (Adjuvant Therapy)**:
    - For women who have undergone **lumpectomy** or **mastectomy**, radiation is often used afterward to kill any remaining cancer cells. Even if no cancer is visible in the breast or nearby areas, radiation can be used to reduce the risk of recurrence.
    - For **lumpectomy patients**, radiation is almost always used to prevent the cancer from coming back in the same breast.

2. **To Shrink Tumors**: In some cases, radiation can be used before surgery (neoadjuvant therapy) to shrink a tumor, making it easier to remove.

3. **For Lymph Node Involvement**: If the cancer has spread to the **lymph nodes** under the arm (axillary

nodes), radiation therapy can help treat the area to reduce the risk of the cancer returning.

4. **For Palliative Care**: In advanced stages of breast cancer, radiation may be used to reduce symptoms such as pain from metastasis (when the cancer spreads to other parts of the body).

How Does Radiation Therapy Work?

Radiation therapy works by damaging the DNA within cancer cells. This damage prevents the cancer cells from growing and dividing, eventually leading to their death. However, normal cells can also be affected by radiation, though they are typically better at repairing themselves than cancer cells.

The radiation is delivered in small doses over a series of sessions to minimize harm to healthy tissue. Each treatment lasts only a few minutes, and the overall course of radiation therapy usually lasts 3 to 7 weeks, depending on the individual case.

The process of receiving radiation therapy generally involves the following steps:

1. **Planning Session**: Before starting treatment, the medical team will conduct a detailed planning session, including imaging tests like a CT scan, to map out exactly where the radiation should be targeted. The goal is to ensure that the radiation is focused on the tumor and not on surrounding healthy tissues.

2. **Treatment Sessions**: Radiation is typically delivered daily (Monday through Friday) for several weeks. Each session is quick and painless, and you will lie on a treatment table while the machine directs radiation to the specific area of the breast.

3. **Follow-up**: After treatment, the doctor will monitor progress and check for any side effects. Regular follow-ups may be necessary to ensure that the cancer has been fully treated.

Possible Side Effects of Radiation Therapy

Like all treatments, radiation therapy can cause side effects, although not everyone experiences them, and they vary in severity. Many side effects are temporary, but some may last longer. Here's an overview of the potential side effects:

Short-Term Side Effects:

1. **Skin Irritation**:
    - The skin in the treated area may become red, dry, itchy, or sensitive, similar to a sunburn. This typically starts a few days to weeks into treatment.
    - The skin may peel or become flaky, but this usually heals after treatment ends. It's important to avoid applying harsh lotions or creams without the doctor's approval.

2. **Fatigue**:
    - Many women report feeling tired or fatigued during radiation therapy. This can affect daily activities but usually improves a few weeks after treatment is completed.

3. **Breast Tenderness or Swelling**:
    - The treated breast may feel swollen or sore, especially if the radiation is directed near the chest wall. This can make wearing tight clothing or a bra uncomfortable.

4. **Pain**:

- If the radiation is targeting the chest wall or lymph nodes, you may experience some soreness or muscle tightness in the treated area.

Long-Term Side Effects:

1. **Changes in Skin Appearance**:
    - Some women experience changes in skin color or texture in the treated area, which may be permanent. Skin may appear darker or slightly thicker.

2. **Lymphedema**:
    - If radiation targets the lymph nodes, it can sometimes cause **lymphedema**, which is swelling in the arm or hand caused by fluid buildup. This is especially common if the axillary lymph nodes are treated.

3. **Heart and Lung Issues**:
    - If radiation is directed near the heart or lungs, there is a small risk of damage to these organs, leading to conditions like heart disease or lung problems. This is more of a concern in left-sided breast cancer treatments, as the heart is located closer to the left breast.

4. **Risk of Second Cancers**:
    - Though rare, radiation therapy can slightly increase the risk of developing a second, different cancer later in life. The risk is more significant in younger patients and depends on factors like the amount of radiation used.

Managing Side Effects

Your healthcare team will work closely with you to manage and minimize side effects. It's important to report any discomfort, pain, or changes you experience during treatment. Here are some general tips for managing radiation side effects:

- **Skin care**: Use mild, unscented lotions to soothe the skin (if approved by your doctor). Wear loose, comfortable clothing to reduce irritation.
- **Rest**: Fatigue is common during radiation, so be sure to rest and take naps when needed.
- **Hydration**: Drink plenty of water to stay hydrated and help your body manage any side effects.
- **Exercise**: Gentle exercise, such as walking, can help reduce fatigue and improve overall well-being.

Chemotherapy

Chemotherapy is one of the most well-known and widely used treatments for breast cancer. It involves the use of powerful drugs to kill cancer cells or stop them from growing and dividing. Chemotherapy can be used alone or in combination with other treatments like surgery, radiation, or hormone therapy, depending on the stage and type of cancer. While chemotherapy is highly effective in treating cancer, it can also affect healthy cells, leading to various side effects.

What Is Chemotherapy?

Chemotherapy refers to the use of **cytotoxic drugs**, which are chemicals designed to destroy or damage cancer cells. These drugs work by targeting cells that are rapidly dividing, which is a hallmark of cancerous cells. However, chemotherapy can also affect normal, healthy cells that divide quickly, such as those in the hair follicles, digestive tract, and bone marrow. This is why chemotherapy often has side effects.

The drugs can be administered in several ways:

- **Intravenously (IV)**: Through a needle inserted into a vein, usually in your arm.
- **Orally**: In the form of pills or capsules that are taken by mouth.
- **Injections**: Sometimes given as an injection under the skin or into a muscle.

Chemotherapy can be given in cycles, with a period of treatment followed by rest, to allow the body time to recover.

When Is Chemotherapy Used?

Chemotherapy is typically used in the following scenarios:

1. **After Surgery (Adjuvant Therapy)**:
    - For women with early-stage breast cancer, chemotherapy may be recommended after surgery to kill any remaining cancer cells that may not be detectable by imaging tests. This helps reduce the risk of the cancer returning.

2. **Before Surgery (Neoadjuvant Therapy)**:
    - In some cases, chemotherapy is given before surgery to shrink a tumor, making it easier to remove. This is often used for larger tumors or aggressive cancers.

3. **For Advanced or Metastatic Cancer**:
    - If breast cancer has spread to other parts of the body (metastatic breast cancer), chemotherapy can be used to control the growth of the cancer and alleviate symptoms.

4. **In Combination with Other Treatments**:
    - Chemotherapy may be used alongside other therapies, like hormone therapy, targeted therapy, or immunotherapy, to increase the chances of treatment success.

How Does Chemotherapy Work?

Chemotherapy works by targeting rapidly dividing cells. Cancer cells grow and divide faster than most healthy cells, making them more susceptible to chemotherapy. However, because chemotherapy drugs are not selective, they can also affect other healthy cells that divide quickly, such as those in the bone marrow, hair follicles, and digestive system.

There are two main mechanisms by which chemotherapy drugs work:

1. **Killing Cancer Cells Directly**: Some chemotherapy drugs directly damage the DNA inside cancer cells, causing them to die or stop growing.

2. **Preventing Cancer Cell Division**: Other chemotherapy drugs stop cancer cells from dividing, preventing them from growing and spreading.

Although chemotherapy does not directly target specific types of breast cancer, it can still be highly effective in reducing the size of the tumor, preventing its spread, or eradicating remaining cancer cells after surgery.

Common Chemotherapy Drugs Used for Breast Cancer

There are many different chemotherapy drugs used for breast cancer, but some of the most common ones include:

1. **Doxorubicin (Adriamycin)**: Often used for aggressive breast cancers. It can be associated with a higher risk of heart problems, so doctors monitor heart health during treatment.
2. **Cyclophosphamide**: Often used in combination with other chemotherapy drugs.
3. **Paclitaxel (Taxol)**: Targets the cancer cells by interfering with their ability to divide and grow.
4. **Docetaxel (Taxotere)**: Similar to paclitaxel, this drug is used to stop cancer cells from dividing.
5. **Fluorouracil (5-FU)**: A drug used to slow the growth of cancer cells.

These drugs can be used alone or in combination with each other, depending on the specific needs of the patient.

Possible Side Effects of Chemotherapy

Because chemotherapy targets all rapidly dividing cells, not just cancer cells, it can cause a range of side effects. The severity of side effects varies depending on the chemotherapy drugs used, the dose, and how the individual responds to treatment. Here's an overview of the most common side effects:

1. Hair Loss (Alopecia)

- One of the most well-known side effects of chemotherapy is hair loss. This happens because chemotherapy targets rapidly dividing cells, including those in hair follicles. Most patients will lose hair on the scalp, and some may lose body hair as well.

- Hair typically begins to fall out 2 to 3 weeks after treatment begins, but it usually grows back once treatment is finished.

2. Fatigue

- Chemotherapy can cause extreme tiredness, known as fatigue. This is a common side effect and can make it difficult to complete everyday activities. Fatigue can last for weeks or months after treatment ends, but it typically improves over time.

3. Nausea and Vomiting

- Many chemotherapy drugs can cause nausea and vomiting. Doctors often prescribe anti-nausea medications to help manage these symptoms. Some people may also experience loss of appetite.

4. Suppressed Immune System (Neutropenia)

- Chemotherapy can weaken the immune system by lowering the number of white blood cells, making patients more susceptible to infections. Your doctor may monitor your blood cell counts and may advise precautions to avoid infection.

5. Mouth Sores

- Some chemotherapy drugs can cause sores or ulcers inside the mouth. This can make eating and drinking painful, and proper oral hygiene is essential to prevent infections.

6. Anemia

- Chemotherapy can lower red blood cell counts, leading to anemia, which causes symptoms like tiredness, shortness of breath, and dizziness.

7. Changes in Menstrual Cycle

- Chemotherapy may cause temporary or permanent changes in the menstrual cycle, and some women may experience menopause as a result of the treatment, especially if they are premenopausal.

8. Peripheral Neuropathy

- Some chemotherapy drugs can cause nerve damage, leading to tingling, numbness, or pain in the hands and feet. This is known as **peripheral neuropathy** and may improve after treatment ends.

9. Diarrhea or Constipation

- Chemotherapy can also affect the digestive system, leading to diarrhea or constipation. Doctors may recommend medications or dietary changes to manage these issues.

Managing Side Effects

While chemotherapy can cause significant side effects, many of them are temporary and manageable. Your healthcare team will closely monitor you during treatment to help minimize side effects and provide supportive care. Some tips to manage side effects include:

- **Stay hydrated**: Drink plenty of fluids to stay hydrated, especially if you are experiencing nausea or diarrhea.

- **Eat small, frequent meals**: Eating small meals throughout the day can help prevent nausea and maintain energy levels.
- **Rest**: Give your body the time it needs to recover by getting plenty of sleep and resting when needed.
- **Hair care**: While hair loss can be emotionally difficult, consider wigs, scarves, or hats as options to help you feel more comfortable.
- **Antibiotics and medications**: If your immune system is weakened, your doctor may prescribe medications to help fight infections or manage symptoms like pain.

Targeted Therapies

In recent years, advancements in cancer treatment have led to the development of **targeted therapies**, which are designed to specifically target and attack cancer cells with greater precision. Unlike traditional chemotherapy, which affects both healthy and cancerous cells, targeted therapies focus on specific molecules or pathways that are involved in the growth and spread of cancer. These therapies are often used in combination with other treatments and have shown great promise in improving the outcomes for many breast cancer patients, especially those with specific types of breast cancer like HER2-positive or BRCA-related cancers.

In this section, we will explore two of the most well-known types of targeted therapies used in breast cancer treatment: **HER2-targeted therapy** and **PARP inhibitors**.

HER2-Targeted Therapy: Targeting the HER2 Protein

Some breast cancers have a mutation in a gene called **HER2** (Human Epidermal growth factor Receptor 2). This gene makes a protein that promotes cell growth. In **HER2-positive breast cancer**, there are too many HER2 proteins on the surface of the cancer cells, which makes the cells grow and divide uncontrollably.

HER2-positive breast cancer tends to be more aggressive, but the good news is that **HER2-targeted therapies** are specifically designed to block this overactive protein, slowing down the growth of the cancer or even eliminating it. These therapies can significantly improve the prognosis for people with HER2-positive breast cancer.

How Does HER2-Targeted Therapy Work?

HER2-targeted therapies work by either blocking the HER2 protein's ability to send growth signals to the cancer cells or by using antibodies that mark the cancer cells for destruction by the immune system. The two main classes of HER2-targeted therapies are:

1. **Monoclonal Antibodies**: These are laboratory-made antibodies that specifically target the HER2 protein. The most widely known monoclonal antibody is **trastuzumab (Herceptin)**. Herceptin binds to the HER2 protein and prevents the cancer cell from receiving growth signals. It can be used alone or in combination with chemotherapy to improve effectiveness.

2. **Small Molecule Inhibitors**: These drugs, such as **lapatinib (Tykerb)**, target HER2 from inside the cell, preventing it from signaling cancer cells to grow. These therapies may be used in combination with other drugs to treat advanced breast cancer.

In many cases, HER2-targeted therapies have been proven to reduce the risk of the cancer returning after surgery (adjuvant therapy) and help shrink tumors before surgery (neoadjuvant therapy). They are also used to treat metastatic breast cancer that has spread to other parts of the body.

Possible Side Effects of HER2-Targeted Therapy

While HER2-targeted therapies can be very effective, they can also cause side effects. Some common side effects include:

- **Heart issues**: Drugs like Herceptin can affect the heart, leading to heart failure or other heart-related complications. Heart function is monitored during treatment.

- **Infusion reactions**: Some patients may experience reactions like fever, chills, or rash when receiving the drug via infusion.

- **Nausea and diarrhea**: These are common with many cancer treatments, including HER2-targeted therapies.

The benefits of HER2-targeted therapies often outweigh the risks, and doctors closely monitor patients to manage any potential side effects.

PARP Inhibitors: Targeting DNA Repair Mechanisms

Another exciting development in targeted therapy is the use of **PARP inhibitors**, particularly for women with breast cancer linked to mutations in the **BRCA1** or **BRCA2** genes. These genes are responsible for repairing damaged DNA in healthy cells. When either of these genes is mutated, the ability to repair DNA is compromised, increasing the likelihood of developing cancer.

PARP (Poly (ADP-Ribose) Polymerase) is an enzyme that helps repair damaged DNA, and **PARP inhibitors** are drugs designed to block this enzyme. By inhibiting PARP, these drugs prevent the repair of DNA damage in cancer cells, leading to the death of these cells, especially in cancers with BRCA mutations, which are already genetically unstable.

How Do PARP Inhibitors Work?

In normal cells, when DNA is damaged, PARP enzymes step in to fix it. However, in cancer cells, particularly those with BRCA1 or BRCA2 mutations, the cancer cells rely on the PARP enzyme to repair their DNA. PARP inhibitors like **olaparib (Lynparza)**, **talazoparib (Talzenna)**, and **niraparib (Zejula)** block the action of PARP, leading to the accumulation of DNA damage and the death of cancer cells.

PARP inhibitors are particularly effective for women with **HER2-negative breast cancer** that carries a BRCA mutation, as these cancers are more likely to respond to treatments that target DNA repair mechanisms.

Possible Side Effects of PARP Inhibitors

PARP inhibitors are generally well-tolerated, but they can cause some side effects, including:

- **Low blood cell counts**: A decrease in red blood cells, white blood cells, or platelets, leading to fatigue, increased risk of infections, or bleeding problems.

- **Nausea and vomiting**: Like many cancer treatments, PARP inhibitors can cause gastrointestinal symptoms.

- **Fatigue**: Many people experience tiredness or lack of energy during treatment.

- **Anemia**: This can lead to symptoms like shortness of breath, dizziness, or pale skin.

Doctors carefully monitor blood counts and overall health during treatment to minimize side effects.

Benefits of Targeted Therapies

The main advantage of targeted therapies, such as **HER2-targeted therapy** and **PARP inhibitors**, is their ability to specifically target cancer cells while minimizing harm to normal, healthy cells. This precision allows for a more **personalized approach** to treatment, which can lead to better outcomes with fewer side effects compared to traditional chemotherapy.

Targeted therapies have improved survival rates, particularly for patients with specific breast cancer subtypes, such as HER2-positive and BRCA-related cancers. By attacking cancer cells at a molecular level, these therapies offer a **more effective** and **less toxic** treatment option, making them an exciting avenue for breast cancer care.

Immunotherapy

Immunotherapy is an innovative and rapidly evolving approach to cancer treatment that aims to **boost or enhance the body's immune system** to recognize and attack cancer cells more effectively. Unlike traditional treatments like chemotherapy and radiation, which target cancer cells directly, immunotherapy works by **stimulating the immune system** to identify and destroy abnormal cells, including cancer cells.

For many years, the body's immune system has been a natural defense against infections, foreign invaders, and even cancer cells. However, cancer cells can sometimes evade detection or suppress the immune system's response, allowing them to grow unchecked. Immunotherapy helps "**unmask**" cancer cells, making them more visible to the immune system, and enables the immune system to fight cancer more effectively.

How Does Immunotherapy Work in Breast Cancer?

Immunotherapy works by targeting different parts of the immune system to increase its ability to fight cancer. There are several ways immunotherapy can be used to treat breast cancer:

Immune Checkpoint Inhibitors:

The immune system has "checkpoint" proteins that act as a sort of "brake" to prevent immune cells from attacking normal cells in the body. Cancer cells can exploit these checkpoints to avoid being attacked by the immune system. **Immune checkpoint inhibitors** work by blocking these brakes, thereby **allowing immune cells (like T-cells)** to recognize and attack cancer cells.

The most common immune checkpoint proteins targeted in breast cancer are **PD-1** and **PD-L1**. By blocking these proteins, **PD-1 inhibitors** such as **pembrolizumab (Keytruda)** and **nivolumab (Opdivo)**, as well as **PD-L1 inhibitors** like **atezolizumab (Tecentriq)**, can help reactivate the immune system's response to cancer. These inhibitors have shown effectiveness particularly in **triple-negative breast cancer** (TNBC), an aggressive form of breast cancer that doesn't respond well to other treatments like hormone therapy or HER2-targeted therapy.

Monoclonal Antibodies:

Monoclonal antibodies are lab-made molecules that can mimic the immune system's ability to fight off harmful pathogens, including cancer. These antibodies can be designed to **target specific cancer cells** directly, helping the immune system to identify and destroy them. For example, **trastuzumab (Herceptin)** is a monoclonal antibody used in

HER2-positive breast cancer, but the concept of monoclonal antibodies extends to immunotherapy, where some are designed to **stimulate the immune system** in addition to targeting cancer cells.

Cancer Vaccines:

While still largely experimental, **cancer vaccines** are designed to stimulate the immune system to recognize and attack cancer cells. These vaccines use specific proteins or antigens found on cancer cells to "teach" the immune system how to identify and target cancer. For breast cancer, vaccines targeting the HER2 protein or other tumor-specific proteins are being explored as a way to prevent recurrence after surgery or chemotherapy.

Adoptive Cell Therapy:

This approach involves **harvesting immune cells** from the patient's own body, enhancing or modifying them in the lab to better recognize and fight cancer cells, and then infusing them back into the patient's body. While this type of therapy is more commonly associated with cancers like leukemia or lymphoma, it holds potential for treating certain breast cancers as well.

Immunotherapy in Breast Cancer: What's the Evidence?

Immunotherapy has become an important treatment option for certain types of breast cancer, particularly for **triple-negative breast cancer (TNBC)** and **HER2-positive breast cancer**. Triple-negative breast cancer, which lacks estrogen, progesterone, and HER2 receptors, is known for being difficult to treat with traditional therapies. However, immune checkpoint inhibitors, such as **atezolizumab (Tecentriq)** in combination with chemotherapy, have shown encouraging results in improving progression-free survival rates for some patients with TNBC.

For **HER2-positive breast cancer**, immunotherapy is also being tested in combination with **HER2-targeted therapies** to further boost treatment effectiveness and reduce the chances of relapse. These therapies help the immune system recognize and attack HER2-overexpressing cells more effectively.

Immunotherapy has been a breakthrough for some patients, offering options when traditional therapies fail or aren't as effective. However, **not all patients respond** to immunotherapy, and research is ongoing to better understand why.

Potential Benefits of Immunotherapy

1. **Durability of Response:** One of the most exciting aspects of immunotherapy is its potential for **long-term effectiveness**. Unlike chemotherapy, which tends to only work for a while before cancer cells become resistant, immunotherapy may help the immune system "remember" the cancer cells and continue to target them long after treatment ends.

2. **Fewer Side Effects:** Since immunotherapy specifically targets cancer cells, it may cause fewer side effects than traditional treatments like chemotherapy and radiation, which can affect both healthy and cancerous cells. The side effects of immunotherapy are often related to an overactive immune response, which can lead to inflammation or autoimmune-like reactions in some patients.

3. **Targeted Action:** Immunotherapy can be **tailored to specific subtypes of breast cancer**, making it possible to treat certain types more effectively than others. This precision leads to more personalized and less invasive treatment options.

Challenges and Side Effects of Immunotherapy

While immunotherapy offers a new hope for breast cancer patients, it's not without its challenges and potential side effects. Some of the common side effects include:

- **Autoimmune-like reactions:** The immune system, once activated, may start attacking healthy tissues as well as cancer cells, leading to inflammation in organs like the lungs, liver, or intestines.
- **Fatigue and flu-like symptoms:** Many patients experience fatigue, fever, or muscle aches during immunotherapy.
- **Skin rashes:** Some immunotherapy drugs can cause skin reactions, including rashes or itchiness.

Additionally, not every patient responds to immunotherapy, and **predicting who will benefit** from this treatment remains a challenge. As a result, ongoing research is focused on identifying biomarkers and developing ways to better predict which patients will benefit from immunotherapy.

Hormone Therapy

Hormone therapy is a common treatment for **hormone receptor-positive** breast cancers—those that grow in response to hormones like **estrogen** and **progesterone**. About **70% of breast cancers** are hormone receptor-positive, meaning that the cancer cells have receptors on their surfaces that bind to these hormones, fueling their growth.

Hormone therapy works by blocking or lowering the levels of these hormones in the body, thereby **slowing or stopping the growth** of the cancer cells. It's a highly effective treatment, especially for women whose cancers are detected at an earlier stage and who are in the **post-menopausal phase**. But how exactly does hormone therapy work, and what are the different treatment options? Let's explore.

How Hormone Therapy Works

Hormones like **estrogen** can fuel the growth of certain types of breast cancer by binding to estrogen receptors (ER) on the cancer cells. **Progesterone** can also play a role in promoting cancer cell growth. Hormone therapy aims to **block the effect of these hormones** on the cancer cells or lower the amount of hormones in the body, making it harder for the cancer to grow.

Hormone therapy can either **block the hormones from attaching to their receptors** (blocking the action of the hormone) or **lower the levels of the hormones** in the body to reduce their availability. There are several approaches to hormone therapy, which can be used alone or in combination with other treatments.

Types of Hormone Therapy for Breast Cancer

Selective Estrogen Receptor Modulators (SERMs)

One of the most common drugs used in hormone therapy is **tamoxifen**. This drug is a **Selective Estrogen Receptor Modulator (SERM)**, which works by **blocking estrogen receptors** on breast cancer cells, preventing estrogen from binding to them. While it doesn't lower estrogen levels in the body, tamoxifen effectively **prevents estrogen** from fueling cancer cell growth.

Tamoxifen is typically used in **premenopausal women** and is often prescribed for **5 to 10 years** after the completion of surgery or other treatments to **lower the risk of recurrence**. It can be used in both early-stage and advanced breast cancer.

Some other SERMs that might be used less frequently include **raloxifene** and **toremifene**, which work in a similar way to tamoxifen.

Aromatase Inhibitors (AIs)

For **postmenopausal women, aromatase inhibitors** are often used. These drugs work by **lowering estrogen production** in the body by blocking the enzyme **aromatase**, which is responsible for turning androgens (hormones like testosterone) into estrogen. By reducing the overall level of estrogen, aromatase inhibitors **starve estrogen receptor-positive cancer cells**, slowing or stopping their growth.

Common aromatase inhibitors include:

- **Letrozole (Femara)**
- **Anastrozole (Arimidex)**
- **Exemestane (Aromasin)**

These medications are usually taken for **5 to 10 years** after surgery, chemotherapy, or radiation to help reduce the risk of recurrence in **early-stage** breast cancer. They are also used to treat **advanced or metastatic** breast cancer.

Ovarian Suppression

In premenopausal women, another approach is **ovarian suppression**, which reduces the amount of estrogen produced by the ovaries. This can be done using surgery, radiation, or medication. Medications like **goserelin (Zoladex)** or **leuprolide (Lupron)** are used to **suppress ovarian function** temporarily, effectively lowering estrogen levels.

Ovarian suppression may be used in combination with **tamoxifen** or an **aromatase inhibitor** in younger women who haven't reached menopause. This approach helps ensure that the cancer cells are no longer able to access estrogen, even if their ovaries are still producing small amounts.

Benefits of Hormone Therapy

1. **Reduces the Risk of Recurrence:** Hormone therapy is effective in **reducing the risk of recurrence** for patients with hormone receptor-positive breast cancer. By preventing estrogen from fueling the growth of remaining cancer cells, hormone therapy lowers the chance of the cancer returning after surgery, radiation, or chemotherapy.

2. **Improved Survival Rates:** Studies have shown that women with hormone receptor-positive breast cancer who receive hormone therapy have **better survival rates** than those who do not. In fact, tamoxifen and aromatase inhibitors have been proven to reduce the likelihood of the cancer coming back by a significant margin.

3. **Targeted Action:** Hormone therapy is **less toxic** than chemotherapy because it specifically targets hormone-sensitive cancer cells, leaving other cells in the body unharmed. This often results in **fewer side effects** compared to traditional treatments like chemotherapy.

Side Effects of Hormone Therapy

While hormone therapy is generally well-tolerated, it can come with a range of **side effects**, some of which can significantly affect a woman's quality of life. Common side effects include:

1. **Hot Flashes:** One of the most common side effects, particularly with **tamoxifen** and **aromatase inhibitors**, is the occurrence of **hot flashes** or night

sweats, which can be quite uncomfortable for some women.

2. **Joint Pain:** Aromatase inhibitors, in particular, can cause **joint pain** or stiffness, which may interfere with daily activities.

3. **Fatigue:** Many women report feeling **tired or fatigued** while on hormone therapy, which can affect both physical and mental well-being.

4. **Mood Swings or Depression:** Hormonal changes caused by treatment can lead to **mood swings**, irritability, and even depression in some women.

5. **Bone Health:** Long-term use of aromatase inhibitors can cause **bone thinning** or **osteoporosis**, increasing the risk of fractures. Doctors often monitor bone health during treatment.

6. **Vaginal Dryness:** Hormone therapy, especially aromatase inhibitors and ovarian suppression, can lead to **vaginal dryness**, which may cause discomfort during intercourse or other related issues.

7. **Increased Risk of Blood Clots: Tamoxifen** can increase the risk of **blood clots** or deep vein thrombosis (DVT), particularly in women with other risk factors.

Duration of Hormone Therapy

The length of hormone therapy can vary depending on the type of breast cancer, the patient's age, and other factors. Typically, **hormone therapy lasts for 5 to 10 years**, with some patients continuing it longer if there is a higher risk of recurrence. Research suggests that longer periods of hormone therapy may offer greater benefits, though the side effects can become more pronounced over time.

Clinical Trials

Clinical trials play a **crucial role** in the fight against breast cancer. These trials are research studies that test new treatments, drugs, therapies, and other medical strategies to determine whether they are safe and effective for patients. By participating in clinical trials, patients not only contribute to **advancing medical knowledge** but may also gain access to **cutting-edge treatments** that aren't available through traditional care routes. For many breast cancer patients, **clinical trials offer hope** for better outcomes and improved quality of life. They provide opportunities to explore **innovative treatments** and sometimes offer access to therapies that are not yet widely available.

What Are Clinical Trials?

Clinical trials are organized studies that **test new medical interventions**, such as:

- **New drugs** or **medications**
- **Surgical procedures** or **techniques**
- **Radiation therapies**
- **Immunotherapies**
- **Combination treatments**

These trials help determine the safety and efficacy of these interventions, compare them with standard treatments, and evaluate the **long-term effects** on patients. Clinical trials are conducted in **phases**:

1. **Phase 1**: The new treatment is tested on a small group of patients for the first time to assess safety, dosage, and side effects.
2. **Phase 2**: The treatment is given to a larger group of patients to evaluate its effectiveness and monitor further side effects.
3. **Phase 3**: The treatment is compared to standard treatments and tested on even larger groups of patients to confirm its efficacy and monitor long-term safety.
4. **Phase 4**: Once a treatment is approved, ongoing studies monitor its long-term effects and effectiveness in larger populations.

Why Are Clinical Trials Important in Breast Cancer Treatment?

1. **Access to Innovative Treatments:** Clinical trials offer patients the chance to receive **cutting-edge therapies** that may not yet be available outside of the study. This is especially important for patients whose cancer hasn't responded well to standard treatments or those who are in advanced stages of breast cancer. Clinical trials may test therapies like **targeted treatments**, **immunotherapies**, or **new chemotherapy drugs** that could provide better outcomes.
2. **Contributing to Medical Progress:** By participating in clinical trials, patients are helping to **advance the science of cancer treatment**. Many of the current therapies that are now common in cancer care were tested first in clinical trials. Without volunteers, it would be difficult to make progress in finding more effective treatments for breast cancer.

3. **Comprehensive Care:** Patients in clinical trials often receive **additional monitoring** and care. The healthcare team in a trial is typically made up of **specialists** who closely follow the patient's progress, provide detailed testing, and offer personalized care plans. This can mean **extra attention** to a patient's overall health.

4. **Possibility of a Better Outcome:** Some patients may experience better results with clinical trial treatments compared to standard care. Trials may test new drugs or therapies that are more effective at targeting cancer cells, leading to better treatment responses and, in some cases, **longer survival rates**.

How to Access Clinical Trials

1. **Talk to Your Doctor:** If you're interested in participating in a clinical trial, the first step is to have an open conversation with your doctor. They can help you understand if you're eligible for a trial based on your **cancer type**, **stage**, **health history**, and **current treatment plan**. Your doctor can also help you weigh the **risks and benefits** of enrolling in a trial and guide you through the selection process.

2. **Search for Clinical Trials:** There are several resources where you can search for clinical trials that are open to participants:

    o **ClinicalTrials.gov**: This is a comprehensive database of clinical trials conducted worldwide. You can search for breast cancer trials by location, phase, and other criteria.

    o **Breast Cancer Organizations**: Many cancer advocacy groups, such as the **American**

Cancer Society or **Breast Cancer Research Foundation**, provide information on available trials and can direct you to specific studies.

- **National Cancer Institute (NCI)**: The NCI also offers a clinical trial search tool for cancer patients. Their website includes details on trials for all types of cancer, including breast cancer.

3. **Eligibility Criteria:** Each clinical trial has **specific eligibility criteria** to determine which patients can participate. These criteria can include the type of breast cancer you have, its stage, your age, general health status, and other factors like previous treatments. These criteria are designed to ensure that the study results are reliable and that patients will be safe during the trial.

4. **Informed Consent:** Before enrolling in a clinical trial, you'll be asked to sign an **informed consent form**. This form explains the **purpose of the study**, the **potential risks**, and the **benefits** of participating. It's important to read this document carefully and ask questions if anything is unclear. Your decision to participate should be fully informed.

Types of Clinical Trials for Breast Cancer

1. **Treatment Trials:** These trials focus on testing new treatments for breast cancer. They may involve **new chemotherapy drugs**, **targeted therapies**, **hormonal treatments**, or **immunotherapies** that are being tested for their effectiveness in treating breast cancer.

2. **Prevention Trials:** Prevention trials explore ways to prevent breast cancer or reduce the risk of developing it in people who have never had breast cancer. For example, they might test medications or lifestyle changes that could lower the risk of developing cancer.

3. **Screening Trials:** These trials are designed to test new methods of detecting breast cancer at an earlier stage. Screening trials might include **new imaging technologies** or tests that could improve early detection and diagnosis.

4. **Quality of Life Trials:** These trials focus on improving the quality of life for breast cancer patients during and after treatment. They might explore ways to reduce side effects, improve physical functioning, or manage emotional challenges that come with the disease and treatment.

Risks and Considerations

While clinical trials offer many potential benefits, they also come with some risks:

- **Unknown side effects**: New treatments may cause side effects that aren't yet known.

- **Time commitment**: Clinical trials often require patients to attend frequent doctor appointments, follow-up visits, and extra tests.

- **Placebo**: In some trials, patients may receive a **placebo** or a treatment that is not the active medication being tested, although this is rare in cancer treatment trials.

- **Uncertain outcomes**: There's no guarantee that the experimental treatment will work or be better than existing therapies.

That said, many trials provide **exceptional care** and closely monitor the patients, minimizing risks where possible.

Chapter 7: Coping with the Diagnosis

Emotional and Psychological Impact

A breast cancer diagnosis can be overwhelming, affecting not just the body but also the **mind** and **emotions**. The journey through breast cancer treatment is not only physically demanding but often filled with intense emotional challenges, from **fear** of the unknown to **anxiety** about treatment outcomes. The impact on mental health is just as significant as the physical aspects, and addressing these emotional and psychological concerns is critical for overall well-being.

Anxiety: The Fear of the Unknown

Anxiety is one of the most common emotional responses to a breast cancer diagnosis. The uncertainty about **treatment** and **prognosis** can create an overwhelming sense of fear. This fear might take many forms, such as:

- **Fear of death**: Worries about the possibility of the cancer being **terminal** or not responding to treatment.

- **Fear of recurrence**: Even after successful treatment, the anxiety about cancer returning can linger.

- **Fear of side effects**: Worries about the physical toll of treatments like chemotherapy, radiation, or surgery, including **nausea**, **fatigue**, and **hair loss**.

It's important to recognize that these feelings are natural, but if they become persistent and start interfering with daily life, **counseling** or **therapy** may be helpful. Cognitive-behavioral therapy (CBT), relaxation techniques, and mindfulness can help patients manage anxiety and regain some sense of control.

Depression: The Weight of a Diagnosis

A breast cancer diagnosis can trigger feelings of **sadness** and **hopelessness**. Depression is more than just a bad mood; it's a profound sense of despair that can interfere with day-to-day activities. Symptoms of depression that may accompany a cancer diagnosis include:

- **Persistent sadness or feelings of emptiness**
- **Loss of interest in activities once enjoyed**
- **Fatigue and difficulty concentrating**
- **Sleep disturbances** (either too much or too little)
- **Feelings of worthlessness or guilt**

Depression is common during cancer treatment and can be a response to both the diagnosis and the physical strain of treatment. It's essential for patients to **acknowledge these feelings** and seek help if they experience depression. Support groups, mental health professionals, and anti-depressant medications (under the guidance of a doctor) can be vital in alleviating the emotional burden.

Body Image Concerns: Coping with Physical Changes

Breast cancer treatment can cause significant changes to a person's physical appearance, which can profoundly affect self-esteem and body image. Some of the most visible changes include:

- **Hair loss** due to chemotherapy
- **Scarring** from surgery (lumpectomy or mastectomy)

- **Changes in breast appearance**, such as loss of shape or size after surgery

For many women, the **loss of a breast** or a change in their physical appearance can lead to feelings of **insecurity** or **loss of femininity**. These body image concerns can further deepen emotional distress.

It's important to remember that these feelings are valid, and coping with them is a personal journey. Here are some strategies that may help:

- **Prosthetics and Reconstruction**: Some patients choose breast reconstruction surgery or wear prosthetic breasts to regain a sense of physical wholeness.

- **Support Groups**: Connecting with other breast cancer patients who understand these struggles can provide emotional relief and a sense of solidarity.

- **Counseling**: Talking to a professional about body image issues can help patients process their feelings and develop healthier perspectives.

- **Celebrating Strength**: Focusing on the strength it takes to fight cancer and recognizing the bravery involved can help shift the focus from appearance to resilience.

Impact on Relationships: Navigating Love and Support

A breast cancer diagnosis can strain relationships, both with **partners** and **family members**. The patient may feel guilty about burdening loved ones, while family and partners may struggle to find the right words or actions to offer support. Some relationships grow stronger through this shared experience, while others may be challenged by emotional or practical pressures.

For couples, it's common for the partner not undergoing treatment to experience feelings of **helplessness** and **frustration**, especially when it comes to caregiving. Open and honest communication, setting aside time for mutual support, and seeking couples counseling can help navigate these challenges.

For those with children, especially young ones, a cancer diagnosis can lead to **difficult conversations**. Explaining the disease in an age-appropriate way, reassuring children that their parent is getting the best care, and seeking professional guidance for family counseling can help everyone cope with the emotional toll.

Coping Strategies: Managing the Emotional Toll

While the emotional and psychological impact of breast cancer is significant, there are numerous strategies to help patients manage these challenges. Here are some coping methods that may help:

- **Mindfulness and Relaxation**: Practicing techniques such as **deep breathing**, **meditation**, and **yoga** can help manage stress and anxiety.

- **Expressive Writing**: Journaling your thoughts and feelings can be a cathartic way to process complex emotions.

- **Social Support**: Staying connected with family and friends provides a sense of community and reassurance. Joining a support group (in person or online) where other breast cancer patients share their experiences can provide emotional comfort.

- **Creative Expression**: Engaging in hobbies like painting, music, or crafting can provide an outlet for emotional release and offer moments of joy amidst treatment.

Seeking Professional Help

If you find that anxiety, depression, or body image issues are becoming difficult to manage, it's important to **reach out for professional help**. Psychologists, counselors, and psychiatrists can offer support through individual or group therapy. Support groups, either in person or online, can connect you with others facing similar emotional challenges.

There are also cancer-specific resources available, such as the **American Cancer Society** and other advocacy groups, which provide **mental health services** and **helplines** to assist patients throughout their journey.

Support Systems

A breast cancer diagnosis can feel isolating, but it's important to remember that **you don't have to face this journey alone**. One of the most crucial elements of navigating the emotional, physical, and psychological challenges of breast cancer is building a strong **support system**. Whether through **family, friends**, or **support groups**, having people who care for you can make a world of difference.

The Role of Family: The Pillars of Love and Care

For many, **family** is the first line of support when it comes to a breast cancer diagnosis. Whether it's a spouse, parents, siblings, or children, family members often serve as the **primary caregivers** and emotional anchors throughout the journey.

1. **Emotional Support**: Having a loved one who listens without judgment, offers reassurance, and provides

a sense of security is priceless. Family members often serve as **a safe haven** for the patient to express fears, frustrations, and hopes.

2. **Caregiving Support**: Family members often take on the responsibility of helping with daily tasks, from **doctor's appointments** to **household chores**. This caregiving support can be a lifeline, especially during times when energy levels are low due to treatment.

3. **Practical Help**: Family often steps in to help with tasks that may seem overwhelming, such as **preparing meals**, **helping with children**, or **providing transportation** to and from treatment.

4. **Sense of Normalcy**: In times of crisis, family can provide a much-needed sense of routine. Sharing meals, watching TV together, or doing simple activities can create a comforting sense of normality amidst the chaos of cancer treatment.

However, while family support is invaluable, it can sometimes be emotionally overwhelming for both the patient and their family members. It's essential to **communicate openly** about needs and boundaries. Sometimes, family members may also need their own support, whether it's talking to a counselor or participating in a support group for caregivers.

The Role of Friends: A Shoulder to Lean On

Friends play an equally important role in a breast cancer patient's support system. While family provides a deep sense of connection, **friends** can offer different kinds of support that might feel less heavy or more easily approachable.

1. **Emotional Lifting**: Friends often offer **fresh perspectives** and moments of lightheartedness. They can help to **distract** from the weight of the

diagnosis with humor, shared memories, and comforting companionship. Sometimes, just having someone to talk to or a friend to share a quiet moment can be incredibly healing.

2. **A Source of Encouragement**: Friends who check in, bring flowers, send cards, or simply remind the patient that they're not forgotten provide **moral support**. Their presence can help the patient feel **validated** and loved.

3. **Practical Help**: Much like family, friends can help with practical tasks. Offering to **run errands**, **pick up groceries**, or even **help with babysitting** can relieve stress and give the patient more time to focus on their health.

4. **Providing Social Connections**: Friends can also help the patient maintain a sense of connection to the outside world. By **inviting the patient to social activities** (even if it's just a low-key coffee date), they help the individual feel **less isolated**.

One of the most important roles friends can play is to **respect boundaries**. If the patient needs space, friends should be understanding and respectful. Offering **consistent check-ins**, rather than overwhelming the patient, can ensure that the support remains positive and helpful.

Support Groups: Connecting with Others Who Understand

Support groups offer a unique and incredibly valuable source of support during a breast cancer journey. These groups, whether in person or online, provide a space where patients can share their experiences with others who are facing similar challenges. Knowing that **others understand exactly what you're going through** can alleviate feelings of isolation and help patients feel less alone.

1. **Shared Experiences**: Hearing from others who have been through or are currently undergoing similar experiences can be both **comforting** and **educational**. Support groups provide a space for members to share practical tips, coping strategies, and treatment experiences.

2. **Emotional Validation**: Talking to people who truly understand the emotional toll of breast cancer can be incredibly cathartic. A support group provides a space where members can express their feelings without fear of judgment, knowing that others can relate.

3. **Psychological Support**: Many support groups are led by **trained facilitators**, such as social workers or psychologists, who are equipped to help patients process their feelings, provide resources, and offer professional guidance on mental health challenges.

4. **Encouragement and Empowerment**: Support groups often focus on **empowering patients** by encouraging self-care, fostering hope, and helping patients feel more in control of their own journey. They remind patients that they are capable of facing whatever challenges come their way.

For many patients, being able to connect with others in similar situations is a huge source of strength. **Online support groups** can be especially helpful for those who may not have access to in-person groups due to geographical location or mobility issues. Sites like the **American Cancer Society** or **Breast Cancer Care** provide a list of trusted support groups and forums.

The Role of Professional Support: Therapy and Counseling

In addition to the support of family, friends, and peers, seeking professional emotional support is often essential during the cancer journey. Therapists, counselors, and psychologists who specialize in cancer care can provide tailored support for emotional and psychological challenges.

1. **Individual Therapy**: Professional therapy can help individuals cope with complex emotions like **fear**, **grief**, or **guilt**. A counselor can help patients process difficult feelings, develop coping mechanisms, and offer strategies to manage the psychological toll of cancer treatment.

2. **Group Therapy**: Group therapy allows individuals to share their experiences in a structured setting while also receiving support from trained professionals. This is particularly useful for those who are looking for emotional support beyond a standard support group.

3. **Caregiver Support**: Family members and caregivers may also benefit from **therapy** or **counseling** to help them navigate their own emotional responses to their loved one's cancer diagnosis. Caregivers often face stress and burnout, and professional support can help them manage these pressures.

Mental Health Resources

The emotional and psychological journey of facing a breast cancer diagnosis is just as important as the physical one. The **mental health** of individuals undergoing treatment or recovering from breast cancer deserves attention, care, and support. Whether it's managing **stress**, **anxiety**, **depression**, or the emotional toll that comes with such a challenging diagnosis, seeking mental health resources can be transformative in the healing process.

Therapy Options: Professional Guidance and Emotional Support

Mental health professionals are trained to help people navigate the emotional complexities of cancer. Therapy offers a space to express fears, process difficult emotions, and develop coping mechanisms. Below are some common therapy options available for breast cancer patients:

Individual Therapy (Psychotherapy)

One-on-one therapy with a trained counselor or therapist offers a private space to explore your thoughts and feelings. A therapist can help with **stress management**, **anxiety reduction**, **coping with uncertainty**, and **grief**. Psychotherapy can also address more complex emotions like **anger**, **fear of recurrence**, or the **emotional impact of physical changes** due to treatment (such as hair loss or changes in body image).

Cognitive Behavioral Therapy (CBT)

CBT is a form of therapy focused on identifying and changing negative thought patterns. It is particularly effective for patients dealing with **anxiety**, **depression**, or **distress** related to cancer. CBT can help individuals cope with emotional setbacks by replacing harmful thoughts with more realistic, positive ones, empowering the patient to regain control over their mental state.

Supportive Psychotherapy

This type of therapy provides **emotional support** and **practical coping strategies** in a non-judgmental, supportive environment. It's a good fit for those who need help processing the emotional weight of a cancer diagnosis, but who are not necessarily experiencing severe mental health disorders. It focuses on **strengthening the person's emotional resilience** and **maintaining a sense of hope**.

Family Therapy

Cancer affects the entire family unit, not just the patient. Family therapy can help loved ones communicate openly about their feelings and concerns, and it allows family members to learn how to best support each other during this challenging time. This therapy can also address any **caregiver burnout** or relationship strain.

Support Groups: Peer Support from Those Who Understand

Support groups provide a unique and powerful resource for patients who feel isolated by their diagnosis. Connecting with others who understand what you are going through can be incredibly comforting and validating. Support groups often provide:

Shared Experiences

Talking with others who are going through similar experiences helps reduce feelings of isolation and loneliness. Patients can share tips, advice, and emotional support, knowing that their peers can truly understand their struggles.

Emotional Validation

Support groups offer a safe space for members to express emotions without fear of judgment. Sometimes, just knowing others feel the same way can relieve anxiety or fear. This connection often fosters feelings of solidarity and community.

Practical Advice

Patients in support groups often share practical tips on how to manage side effects of treatment, how to handle certain aspects of care, or how to talk to children and family members about cancer. Support groups can be a valuable resource for sharing strategies and coping techniques.

Online Support Groups

If you prefer more privacy or cannot attend in-person groups, online support groups are an excellent option. There are many dedicated forums, social media groups, and cancer organization sites that provide virtual communities where patients can connect from the comfort of their own home.

Caregiver Support Groups

It's not only the patient who needs support. Caregivers can also benefit from attending support groups designed for those taking care of someone with breast cancer. These groups provide a space for caregivers to share their struggles, receive emotional support, and learn how to manage the stresses of caregiving.

Mindfulness Techniques: Cultivating Inner Peace and Emotional Balance

In addition to therapy and support groups, **mindfulness techniques** can be incredibly helpful in managing stress and maintaining emotional balance during breast cancer treatment. Mindfulness involves focusing on the present moment with **acceptance** and **awareness**, which can reduce feelings of anxiety, depression, and emotional overwhelm. Here are some mindfulness techniques to try:

Mindfulness Meditation

Mindfulness meditation involves focusing your attention on your breath or a specific word or phrase (mantra) while letting go of distracting thoughts. This simple practice can be calming and help patients manage stress, as well as improve their overall sense of well-being. Even just a few minutes a day can reduce **stress** and increase **emotional resilience**.

Deep Breathing Exercises

Deep breathing techniques help activate the body's **relaxation response**, lowering stress and anxiety. A common technique is **diaphragmatic breathing**, which involves breathing deeply through your abdomen (rather than your chest). By slowing down the breath, this technique promotes calmness and can be especially useful during treatment or stressful moments.

Guided Imagery

Guided imagery is a relaxation technique where you visualize a peaceful place or situation, such as a beach or a forest, to help promote calm. This technique has been shown to reduce **anxiety**, improve **mood**, and enhance the body's healing abilities by reducing stress levels.

Yoga and Tai Chi

Both **yoga** and **tai chi** are gentle, low-impact exercises that incorporate mindfulness and movement. These practices help improve flexibility, reduce stress, and provide a mental break. Yoga, in particular, focuses on **breathing**, **body awareness**, and **gentle stretching**, which can help alleviate both physical and emotional tension.

Journaling

Writing down your thoughts and feelings can be a great way to process emotions. Journaling provides a safe space to express yourself and can help you reflect on your emotional journey, track your healing progress, and set personal goals. It can also be an outlet for managing feelings of frustration or fear.

Combining Resources for Better Mental Health

The key to a successful mental health strategy during breast cancer treatment is combining **multiple resources** to address your emotional and psychological well-being. Therapy offers professional guidance, support groups provide shared experiences and emotional validation, and mindfulness techniques help manage stress and anxiety. By using a combination of these approaches, you can build a **holistic support system** that nurtures your emotional health during every phase of your breast cancer journey.

It's essential to remember that taking care of your mind is just as important as taking care of your body. By prioritizing your mental health, you will be better equipped to cope with the challenges of cancer and ultimately find **peace, strength, and resilience** in your journey.

Life After Treatment

Reaching the end of active breast cancer treatment is a major milestone, but it's just the beginning of a new phase of life. For many patients, the transition to post-treatment can feel both **relieving** and **overwhelming**. While there's a sense of accomplishment, there are also new challenges to face—especially managing the **fear of recurrence** and adjusting to life after treatment.

Follow-Up Care: Ensuring Continued Health and Monitoring

Even after active treatment ends, **ongoing care** is critical to monitor your recovery and ensure the cancer doesn't return. **Follow-up care** is designed to check for any signs of recurrence, monitor your physical health, and address any long-term side effects of treatment. Here's what you can expect:

1. **Regular Check-ups**

    Follow-up visits to your oncologist are typically scheduled every **3 to 6 months** in the first few years after treatment, and then less frequently as time passes. These check-ups are essential for catching any signs of cancer returning, and for addressing concerns or side effects that may emerge after treatment. Your doctor will monitor your health through **physical exams**, ask about any symptoms or changes you've noticed, and conduct routine tests.

2. **Imaging Tests and Blood Work**

    Depending on your individual situation, your doctor may recommend imaging tests, such as **mammograms**, **ultrasound**, or **MRI** scans. These tests are used to monitor your breast health and check for any changes that could suggest the cancer has returned. Blood tests may also be used to look for tumor markers or other signs of recurrence. These tests help detect cancer early if it does return, giving you the best chance for effective treatment.

3. **Managing Long-Term Side Effects**

    Breast cancer treatments like chemotherapy, radiation, and surgery can leave long-term side effects, including fatigue, joint pain, neuropathy (nerve pain), changes in skin texture, or even issues related to heart health. Your doctor will work with you to manage these ongoing symptoms and improve your quality of life. This may include **physical therapy**, medication for pain relief, or **counseling** to address any emotional toll left by the treatments.

4. **Survivorship Care Plan**

A **survivorship care plan** is a personalized blueprint that your oncologist may provide to guide your post-treatment care. This plan outlines what tests or treatments you should have, how often to follow up with healthcare providers, and recommendations for lifestyle changes to help keep you healthy. The goal of this plan is to give you clear directions for maintaining your health and wellness after cancer treatment.

Managing the Fear of Recurrence: Coping with Uncertainty

After finishing treatment, one of the most common challenges many breast cancer survivors face is the **fear of recurrence**. This fear can be overwhelming and affect your emotional well-being. It's important to acknowledge that while fear is a normal reaction, it doesn't have to control your life. Here are some ways to manage the fear of recurrence:

1. **Acknowledge Your Feelings**

    It's completely normal to feel anxious or fearful about the possibility of cancer returning. Understanding that these feelings are a natural part of the process can help you face them without shame. Talking about your concerns with your healthcare provider, friends, family, or a therapist can provide comfort and reassurance.

2. **Focus on What You Can Control**

    Although you can't control the future, there are things you can do to improve your health and reduce your risk of recurrence. Following your survivorship care plan, eating a healthy diet, exercising, managing stress, and staying up-to-date with screenings and tests are all ways to take charge of your health and well-being. Living a healthy lifestyle may also contribute to a better sense of control and peace of mind.

3. **Mindfulness and Relaxation**

   Techniques like **meditation**, **yoga**, or **deep breathing** can help reduce the anxiety associated with the fear of recurrence. These mindfulness practices are designed to bring your focus to the present moment, which can help you avoid spiraling into fear or negative thoughts about the future. Staying connected to your emotions and allowing yourself to experience them fully without judgment can also help lessen anxiety.

4. **Support Systems**

   Leaning on your **support network** is key. Talking with other cancer survivors can provide perspective and support, as they understand what you're going through. Support groups (either in-person or online) can offer reassurance and a space to express your fears. If necessary, consider speaking with a mental health professional, as therapy can be invaluable in processing the anxiety that comes with the fear of recurrence.

5. **Reframing the Fear**

   For some, transforming the fear into motivation can be empowering. Instead of focusing on the worst-case scenario, try to shift your mindset toward living your best life, appreciating every moment, and staying vigilant about your health. While it's natural to feel fear, learning to **reframe it** and focus on positivity can help lessen its hold over you.

6. **Accepting Uncertainty**

One of the most powerful ways to cope with the fear of recurrence is to accept the uncertainty of life. While it's true that a recurrence may occur, it's equally true that you are living with strength, resilience, and the tools to fight should it happen. Embracing the unknown and accepting that you have **no control over everything** can be a freeing and empowering mindset.

Embracing Life After Treatment: Moving Forward with Hope

Life after breast cancer treatment may bring its share of challenges, but it also opens the door to new possibilities. **Healing**, both physically and emotionally, is a journey, and it's important to approach it with **patience** and **self-compassion**. Whether it's starting new hobbies, spending more time with loved ones, or pursuing long-held dreams, the post-treatment phase offers an opportunity for **renewed focus** and **purpose**.

By prioritizing **follow-up care**, managing the fear of recurrence, and using available mental health resources, you can embrace life after treatment with confidence. Remember, you are not defined by cancer, and every day is a new opportunity to live fully and with hope.

Chapter 8: Nutrition and Lifestyle During Treatment

Dietary Considerations

A healthy diet plays an essential role in supporting your body through breast cancer treatment. Nutrition is not only vital for maintaining energy levels but can also help **manage side effects** like **nausea, fatigue**, and **changes in taste** that often accompany cancer therapies.

The Importance of Nutrients: Fueling Your Body for Recovery

During breast cancer treatment, your body needs more **energy** and **nutrients** to cope with the stress of treatment and to aid in the healing process. Here are some key nutrients and why they're important:

1. **Protein**

    Protein is crucial for repairing tissue and building a strong immune system. After surgery or during chemotherapy, protein helps the body recover and maintain muscle mass. Foods rich in protein include **chicken, fish, eggs, tofu, beans**, and **low-fat dairy products**. If you struggle with eating solid foods, protein shakes or smoothies can provide an easy-to-digest source of protein.

2. **Carbohydrates**

    Carbohydrates are the body's main energy source, and they're essential for keeping your strength up. Whole grains like **brown rice, quinoa**, and **whole-wheat pasta** provide fiber, which is important for digestion, especially if you're experiencing side effects like constipation from treatment. Sweet potatoes, fruits, and vegetables also provide natural sugars and are rich in vitamins and minerals.

3. **Healthy Fats**

   Healthy fats, found in foods like **avocados**, **nuts**, **seeds**, and **olive oil**, help maintain your energy levels and support your body's ability to absorb certain vitamins, like vitamins A, D, and E. These fats also help with inflammation control, which is especially important during cancer treatment.

4. **Vitamins and Minerals**

   Nutrient-rich foods can help support your immune system and overall health. Foods rich in **vitamin C** (like citrus fruits, strawberries, and bell peppers) can help fight infections and boost your body's natural defenses. **Vitamin D** (from sources like **salmon**, **fortified milk**, and sunlight) is important for bone health, especially if you're undergoing chemotherapy, which can affect bone density. **Iron** is also critical, especially if you're feeling fatigued, as it helps carry oxygen in your blood. Iron-rich foods include **spinach**, **red meat**, **beans**, and **lentils**.

Managing Treatment Side Effects: Adjusting Your Diet to Feel Better

Cancer treatments like chemotherapy, radiation, and surgery can cause a range of side effects that make eating more challenging. Here are some tips to help manage common side effects through your diet:

1. **Nausea**

Nausea is a common side effect of chemotherapy and can make eating feel like a struggle. Here are some dietary strategies to help manage nausea:

- **Eat smaller, more frequent meals**: Eating small meals throughout the day instead of three large ones can help ease nausea.

- **Avoid strong smells**: Strong odors can worsen nausea. Stick to bland, easy-to-digest foods like **crackers**, **plain rice**, **applesauce**, or **boiled potatoes**.

- **Ginger**: This natural remedy is known to help with nausea. Try sipping **ginger tea** or nibbling on **ginger candies**.

- **Stay hydrated**: Sip on clear fluids like water, **broth**, or **herbal teas**. Avoid sugary drinks that may exacerbate nausea.

2. **Fatigue**

Many cancer patients experience fatigue due to the physical toll of treatment. Eating the right foods can help maintain your energy:

- **Complex carbs**: Foods like **oatmeal, whole grains**, and **sweet potatoes** release energy slowly, helping to sustain you throughout the day.

- **Protein**: Ensuring that your meals include enough protein can keep you feeling fuller for longer, helping to combat tiredness between meals.

- **Hydration**: Dehydration can worsen fatigue, so it's essential to drink enough water throughout the day. Herbal teas or smoothies can help boost hydration while providing extra nutrients.

3. **Taste Changes**

   Many people undergoing chemotherapy experience changes in taste, including a metallic or bitter taste. This can make eating less enjoyable. To combat this:

   - **Use herbs and spices**: Flavoring your food with **garlic**, **ginger**, **cinnamon**, and **fresh herbs** can help mask any off-tastes and make food more appealing.

   - **Avoid acidic foods**: Foods like **tomatoes** or **citrus** might be less tolerable if you're experiencing a metallic taste. Opt for milder options like **sweet fruits** or **cooked vegetables**.

   - **Experiment with temperature**: Sometimes, cold or room-temperature foods are easier to tolerate than hot meals. Try **cold smoothies**, **yogurt**, or **salads**.

4. **Loss of Appetite**

   A loss of appetite can be caused by many factors, including treatment side effects or emotional stress. To combat this:

   - **Focus on nutrient-dense foods**: If your appetite is low, try to make every bite count by choosing foods high in nutrients, such as **smoothies, protein bars**, and **high-calorie snacks**.

   - **Try liquid meals**: If solid foods are unappealing, liquid options like **soups, smoothies**, and **shakes** can help you get the calories and nutrients you need.

- **Eat favorite comfort foods**: Sometimes, eating something familiar and comforting can help improve your appetite. Consider your favorite foods and don't be afraid to indulge in a small treat.

Staying Nourished During Treatment: Practical Tips

1. **Plan Ahead**

   Preparing meals in advance can help take the stress out of mealtimes, especially when you're feeling fatigued. Batch-cooking soups, casseroles, or smoothies can ensure you have something nutritious ready to go when you need it.

2. **Work with a Nutritionist**

   A **registered dietitian** or nutritionist can be invaluable in helping you create a meal plan that supports your treatment. They can offer advice on managing side effects, suggest supplements, and make sure you're getting the right balance of nutrients.

3. **Stay Flexible**

   Treatment can affect your appetite and food preferences day by day. Be gentle with yourself and adjust as needed. If you don't feel like eating a full meal, opt for something light that you can manage. The most important thing is to **nourish your body** in whatever way works best for you on any given day.

Exercise

Exercise might be the last thing on your mind when dealing with the physical and emotional toll of breast cancer treatment, but moderate physical activity can be one of the most effective ways to improve your well-being during this time. The idea of exercising while undergoing treatment may seem daunting, but it's important to know that even small amounts of exercise can have a **big impact** on both your **physical health** and **mental well-being**.

The Benefits of Moderate Exercise During Treatment

1. **Boosting Energy Levels**

    It might sound counterintuitive, but engaging in light exercise can actually **reduce fatigue** and increase your energy levels. Treatment side effects, particularly chemotherapy, can leave you feeling tired and drained, but studies have shown that moderate exercise, like **walking**, **yoga**, or **swimming**, helps combat this fatigue by improving circulation and promoting better sleep.

2. **Managing Stress and Anxiety**

    A cancer diagnosis can be overwhelming, and the treatments themselves can add stress and anxiety. Exercise has long been proven to help release **endorphins**, the body's natural mood boosters. A brisk walk or a gentle workout can help calm your mind and improve your mood, making it easier to cope with the emotional challenges of cancer treatment.

3. **Improving Muscle Strength and Flexibility**

    Cancer treatments like chemotherapy and radiation can cause muscle weakness and stiffness. Exercise helps maintain **muscle strength** and **flexibility**, which is essential for maintaining mobility and preventing further injury. Strength training and gentle stretching exercises can also help you stay active and prevent the aches and pains that often accompany treatment.

4. **Enhancing Immune Function**

    Regular exercise can help **boost the immune system**, making your body better equipped to fight infections, which is particularly important during breast cancer treatment when your immune system may be weakened. Even low-intensity exercises like walking can promote better circulation, allowing your immune cells to work more effectively.

5. **Helping with Weight Management**

    Weight gain or loss is a common side effect of breast cancer treatment, and exercise can help you maintain a healthy weight or manage any unwanted changes. Combining **strength training** with **cardiovascular** exercise can help regulate your metabolism and improve your overall health.

6. **Promoting Better Sleep**

    Insomnia and disrupted sleep are common during cancer treatment. Exercise can help improve the quality of your sleep by promoting relaxation and reducing anxiety. Just be mindful not to exercise too close to bedtime, as that can make it harder to fall asleep.

Exercise and Recovery: Benefits Post-Treatment

Once your active treatment has ended, incorporating exercise into your daily routine can help speed up recovery and improve overall health. Here's how exercise supports your recovery journey:

1. **Faster Recovery and Healing**

After surgery or chemotherapy, exercise plays a crucial role in **rehabilitation**. It helps improve blood circulation, which is vital for healing, as it delivers essential nutrients to the tissues that need to repair. Additionally, exercise strengthens the heart and lungs, which is essential after the strain treatment puts on these organs.

2. **Reducing the Risk of Recurrence**

    Research shows that regular exercise after breast cancer treatment may **lower the risk of cancer recurrence**. Physical activity helps regulate hormones like estrogen, which plays a role in the development of some breast cancers. Exercise also helps improve the health of your cells and tissue, reducing inflammation and promoting overall wellness.

3. **Improving Mental Health**

    Life after cancer treatment can come with a host of emotional challenges, including **fear of recurrence** and adjusting to a new normal. Exercise provides a sense of accomplishment and can help fight off feelings of **depression, anxiety**, and **stress**. Engaging in activities like yoga or swimming can also be meditative, allowing you to clear your mind and regain a sense of peace.

4. **Strengthening Bones**

    Some cancer treatments, particularly chemotherapy and hormone therapies, can affect bone density, leading to a higher risk of fractures and osteoporosis. Weight-bearing exercises, such as **walking, jogging,** or **strength training**, are essential for improving bone health and lowering the risk of fractures after treatment.

Safe Exercise During Treatment: How to Get Started

While exercise is highly beneficial, it's important to approach it safely, especially during treatment. Here are some tips for exercising during and after treatment:

1. **Start Slow**

    If you've been sedentary or have had long periods of rest, start with low-impact exercises and gradually increase the intensity. A 10- to 20-minute walk can be a great place to start, and as you feel more comfortable, you can extend the duration or increase the pace.

2. **Listen to Your Body**

    It's crucial to pay attention to how your body feels. If you're feeling fatigued or unwell, rest. Don't push yourself too hard. It's okay to take a break and resume your workout when you feel ready.

3. **Consult Your Doctor**

    Before beginning any exercise program, it's important to check with your oncologist or healthcare provider to make sure you're exercising safely, especially if you have complications or concerns specific to your treatment.

4. **Focus on Fun, Low-Impact Activities**

    Find an activity you enjoy to help keep you motivated. Walking, cycling, swimming, or dancing are fun ways to stay active without putting too much strain on your body. **Yoga** and **tai chi** are also great options for improving flexibility and mental well-being, as they combine gentle movement with mindfulness.

5. **Stay Hydrated**

Dehydration can make you feel worse during treatment, so make sure to drink plenty of water before, during, and after exercise. Staying hydrated will help maintain your energy levels and prevent unnecessary fatigue.

Supplements

When undergoing breast cancer treatment and recovery, many individuals seek ways to enhance their overall health and well-being. One option that often comes up is **supplements**—vitamins, minerals, and other nutrients that claim to support the body during this challenging time. But while supplements can offer potential benefits, it's important to approach them with caution and to consult a healthcare provider before incorporating them into your routine.

The Role of Supplements During Cancer Recovery

Cancer treatment often places significant stress on the body. Whether it's surgery, chemotherapy, radiation, or hormone therapy, the body requires extra **nutrients** to help rebuild and recover. Supplements can help fill in the nutritional gaps created by the side effects of treatment, and in some cases, they may offer added support for your immune system and general health. Here's how specific types of supplements might be beneficial during recovery:

1. **Boosting Nutrient Intake**

    Chemotherapy, for example, can cause **nausea, vomiting,** and changes in appetite, making it difficult to get the necessary vitamins and minerals from food alone. In these cases, **multivitamins** or individual nutrients like **vitamin D**, **calcium**, and **B vitamins** can help support overall health by filling nutritional gaps.

2. **Supporting Immune Health**

   Some supplements, such as **vitamin C**, **zinc**, and **probiotics**, may help boost your immune system. This is especially important after cancer treatments, which can weaken immune function. These supplements can help your body fend off infections and stay strong.

3. **Managing Side Effects**

   Some treatments can lead to specific side effects like **dry skin**, **fatigue**, and **joint pain**. Certain supplements, such as **omega-3 fatty acids** (found in fish oil), can help reduce inflammation, while **biotin** and **vitamin E** may promote healthier skin and hair.

4. **Supporting Bone Health**

   Treatments like chemotherapy and hormone therapy can affect bone density, making bones weaker and more prone to fractures. Supplements like **calcium**, **vitamin D**, and **magnesium** are often recommended to help maintain bone health and reduce the risk of osteoporosis.

5. **Improving Energy and Vitality**

   Fatigue is one of the most common side effects of cancer treatments, and it can persist even after treatment ends. Supplements such as **iron** or **B-complex vitamins** may help boost energy levels, particularly if there is an underlying deficiency in these nutrients.

What to Keep in Mind When Considering Supplements

While supplements can be beneficial, they are not a one-size-fits-all solution. Here are some important considerations to keep in mind before adding any supplements to your routine:

1. **Consult Your Doctor First**

   The most important thing to remember is to always **consult with your doctor** or oncologist before taking any new supplements. Your healthcare provider can help determine if supplements are appropriate for you, considering your specific health status, cancer treatment plan, and potential interactions with medications you may be taking.

2. **Interactions with Treatment**

   Some supplements can interfere with cancer treatments or other medications. For example, high doses of **vitamin E** or **green tea extract** might interact with chemotherapy drugs and reduce their effectiveness. Similarly, some supplements, like **garlic** or **ginseng**, can have blood-thinning effects that may be dangerous during surgery or chemotherapy.

3. **Quality and Purity**

   Not all supplements are created equal. It's crucial to choose supplements that are **high-quality** and **free from contaminants**. Always look for brands that are **certified by third-party organizations** for quality and purity. Supplements that aren't regulated by health authorities may not contain the ingredients they claim, or could contain harmful substances.

4. **Whole Foods First**

   While supplements can support your recovery, they should not replace a healthy, balanced diet. Focus on getting most of your nutrients from **whole foods** like fruits, vegetables, lean proteins, and whole grains. Supplements are meant to **complement** your diet, not substitute for it.

5. **Monitor for Side Effects**

   Just like any medication, supplements can have **side effects**, particularly if taken in high doses. Keep track of how your body responds to any new supplement. If you notice any negative effects like nausea, dizziness, or digestive issues, stop taking the supplement and talk to your doctor.

Popular Supplements for Cancer Recovery

Here are some supplements that are commonly used during cancer recovery, but again, always discuss their use with your doctor first:

- **Vitamin D**: Supports bone health, immune function, and overall well-being.

- **Calcium**: Essential for maintaining strong bones, particularly important during and after hormone therapy or chemotherapy.

- **Omega-3 Fatty Acids**: Found in fish oil or flaxseed oil, omega-3s help reduce inflammation and support heart health.

- **Probiotics**: Beneficial for gut health, especially if you're experiencing digestive issues as a result of treatment.

- **Vitamin C**: An antioxidant that supports the immune system and helps the body recover from stress.

- **Iron**: Especially important if you experience fatigue or have anemia due to chemotherapy or blood loss.

- **Turmeric (Curcumin)**: Known for its anti-inflammatory properties, though it's important to check with your doctor due to potential interactions with medications.

Weight Management, Diet, and Fasting

During breast cancer treatment, changes in weight are common, and many people experience either **weight gain** or **weight loss**. These changes can occur due to a variety of factors, including **medications**, **hormonal treatments**, **side effects of chemotherapy or radiation**, and changes in appetite. Managing your weight during this time is important, not only to help you feel your best but also to maintain **overall health** and **well-being**.

Common Weight Changes During Treatment

1. Weight Gain

    - **Hormonal Changes**: Many breast cancer treatments, particularly **hormone therapy** (like Tamoxifen or aromatase inhibitors), can cause **weight gain**. These drugs block estrogen, which can lead to changes in metabolism and fat distribution. This weight gain often occurs around the **abdomen** and **waist**.

    - **Chemotherapy**: While chemotherapy can lead to **nausea** and a loss of appetite, it can also cause some people to gain weight. This may be due to a variety of factors like **fluid retention**, changes in taste or cravings, or a less active lifestyle during treatment.

    - **Reduced Physical Activity**: Feeling fatigued or experiencing side effects like nausea or pain can result in **less physical activity**, which can contribute to weight gain.

2. Weight Loss

- **Loss of Appetite**: Some people experience a reduced appetite due to chemotherapy side effects like **nausea** or **taste changes**. This can make it difficult to maintain a healthy weight.

- **Digestive Issues**: Chemotherapy and radiation therapy may cause gastrointestinal problems like **diarrhea**, **mouth sores**, or **difficulty swallowing**, which can lead to weight loss if nutrition becomes harder to maintain.

- **Increased Metabolism**: In some cases, cancer treatments can increase the body's metabolism, causing you to burn calories faster than usual. This can also lead to unintended weight loss.

Managing Weight Changes During Treatment

Managing your weight during breast cancer treatment requires a balanced approach that focuses on **healthy eating**, **physical activity**, and, if necessary, adjusting your diet to support your body's changing needs.

1. Nutrition: Focus on Whole, Nutrient-Dense Foods

Regardless of whether you are gaining or losing weight, **nutrition** is crucial during cancer treatment. A well-balanced diet supports your immune system, helps repair damaged cells, and gives you the energy you need to feel better. Here are some tips:

- For Weight Gain:

  - **Choose nutrient-dense, calorie-rich foods**: Focus on eating foods that are rich in nutrients but also high in healthy calories.

Good examples include **avocados**, **nuts**, **seeds**, **full-fat dairy**, **olive oil**, and **whole grains**.

- **Balance your macronutrients**: Make sure to include plenty of **protein** (like lean meats, tofu, and legumes) to support muscle repair, as well as **healthy fats** (from sources like nuts, seeds, and fish) and **complex carbohydrates** (from vegetables and whole grains) for sustained energy.

- **Monitor portion sizes**: Eating smaller, more frequent meals throughout the day can help if you're experiencing nausea or a reduced appetite.

- For Weight Loss:

    - **Focus on high-calorie, high-protein meals**: If you are losing weight, try to add **protein-rich** foods like **chicken**, **fish**, **eggs**, **beans**, and **protein shakes** to help maintain muscle mass and promote recovery.

    - **Smoothies**: These are great for people who have trouble eating solid food. You can blend fruits, vegetables, protein powder, and healthy fats (like nut butter or flaxseed oil) to create a calorie-dense meal.

    - **Eat smaller meals more often**: Eating small meals 5-6 times per day can help if you're struggling with a reduced appetite or nausea.

2. Exercise: Move When You Can

While treatment may leave you feeling tired, **exercise** (even moderate exercise) can help manage weight, reduce fatigue, and improve overall quality of life. Some benefits of staying active during treatment include:

- **Preventing Weight Gain**: Regular physical activity can help prevent the kind of weight gain that sometimes accompanies cancer treatment, especially if you're on hormone therapy.

- **Improving Metabolism**: Exercise can support a healthy metabolism, which may help your body process and use nutrients more efficiently.

- **Boosting Mental Health**: Exercise is also known to have positive effects on mood and mental well-being, which is essential when managing the emotional aspects of cancer treatment.

3. Fasting and Weight Management: A Growing Area of Interest

Fasting, or temporarily restricting food intake, has become a topic of growing interest in cancer treatment and recovery. Research into **fasting** and its effects on cancer is still ongoing, but there are some potential benefits to consider:

- **Weight Loss Support**: For those struggling with weight gain during cancer treatment, intermittent fasting (e.g., eating only within a specific window each day) may help regulate calorie intake and encourage weight loss. It may also support improved insulin sensitivity and fat metabolism.

- **Cellular Repair**: Some studies suggest that fasting may help promote cellular repair and **autophagy** (the process by which the body breaks down and recycles damaged cells), which could be beneficial during cancer treatment recovery. However, more research is needed in this area to fully understand its effects.

- **Hormonal Regulation**: Fasting may influence **hormonal balance** and support weight management by helping regulate insulin and estrogen levels. For people who are undergoing hormone therapy, this could potentially have some benefits.

However, **fasting is not recommended for everyone**, and it's crucial to consult with your healthcare team before considering fasting or any dietary changes, especially during active cancer treatment. Your doctor can help determine if fasting could be beneficial, considering your individual treatment plan and nutritional needs.

Chapter 9: The Latest Advances in Research

Personalized Medicine

The era of **personalized medicine** marks an exciting shift in cancer treatment, where therapies are tailored specifically to an individual's genetic makeup, tumor characteristics, and molecular profile. In the case of **breast cancer**, this means that doctors are moving away from a "one-size-fits-all" approach and offering treatments that are uniquely suited to each patient's condition. This customization improves the effectiveness of treatment, reduces side effects, and increases the chances of better outcomes.

What is Personalized Medicine?

Personalized medicine, sometimes called **precision medicine**, refers to the use of genetic, molecular, and clinical information to select treatments that are most likely to be effective for each patient. In the past, treatments were based on broad categories, such as the type of cancer (e.g., breast cancer). However, as research has progressed, doctors have learned that even cancers within the same category can differ dramatically on a molecular level.

Personalized medicine focuses on identifying the specific genetic and molecular features of a patient's cancer. These insights guide doctors in selecting therapies that target those features, ensuring the treatment works more effectively with fewer side effects.

How Does Genetic and Molecular Testing Work?

Genetic and molecular testing involves analyzing both the patient's **tumor** and **blood samples** to identify mutations, biomarkers, and other molecular factors that can influence how the cancer behaves and responds to treatment.

1. Tumor Genetic Testing

The first step in personalizing breast cancer treatment is to test the tumor itself. This may include:

- **Genetic Mutations**: Certain mutations in the tumor's DNA, such as **HER2 overexpression** or mutations in **BRCA genes**, can make the cancer more aggressive or more sensitive to specific treatments.

- **Receptor Status**: Testing whether the tumor expresses **hormone receptors** (like **estrogen** or **progesterone**) or if it overproduces the **HER2 protein** can help determine whether hormone therapy or **HER2-targeted therapy** might be effective.

- **Molecular Profiling**: This can help doctors understand the specific pathways driving the cancer's growth, which could suggest the use of drugs that target those pathways.

2. Liquid Biopsy

A newer, less invasive test, **liquid biopsy**, analyzes a blood sample for genetic material shed by tumors (circulating tumor DNA). This can provide valuable insights into the genetic profile of a cancer and help doctors track how it's evolving throughout treatment.

3. Comprehensive Genomic Profiling

Some cancer centers use more comprehensive tests that look at the full genetic makeup of the tumor, not just a few key markers. This helps doctors identify rare mutations or vulnerabilities in the tumor that might not be obvious from traditional tests.

Types of Personalized Treatments

Based on the results of genetic and molecular tests, breast cancer treatment can be tailored in several ways:

1. Targeted Therapy

Targeted therapies are designed to attack specific molecules that help tumors grow. For example:

- **HER2-targeted therapies** like **trastuzumab (Herceptin)** specifically target HER2-positive tumors, which are found in about 20% of breast cancers. These drugs work by blocking the HER2 protein or preventing it from signaling tumor growth.

- **PARP inhibitors** may be used for people with **BRCA mutations**, as these drugs can prevent cancer cells from repairing their DNA, causing the cells to die off.

2. Hormone Therapy

If a tumor is **hormone receptor-positive**, meaning it grows in response to estrogen or progesterone, hormone therapy can block these hormones or reduce their levels in the body, slowing or stopping cancer growth. Common hormone therapies include **tamoxifen** and **aromatase inhibitors**. Genetic testing can help determine if a patient is likely to benefit from these therapies.

3. Immunotherapy

For some breast cancers, especially **triple-negative breast cancer**, immunotherapy may be used. These treatments help the immune system recognize and attack cancer cells more effectively. Molecular testing can identify tumors that may be more responsive to immunotherapy drugs.

4. Chemotherapy Sensitivity Testing

Certain molecular markers can predict how well a patient will respond to chemotherapy. By analyzing the tumor's specific genetic makeup, doctors can better determine which chemotherapy drugs are most likely to be effective.

Benefits of Personalized Medicine

Personalized medicine has revolutionized the way doctors approach breast cancer treatment. The benefits include:

- **Increased Effectiveness**: By targeting specific mutations or receptors, treatments are more likely to be effective against the cancer, reducing the risk of recurrence.

- **Reduced Side Effects**: Targeted therapies and drugs chosen based on genetic testing tend to cause fewer side effects than traditional chemotherapy, which can affect healthy cells as well as cancer cells.

- **Smarter Treatment Decisions**: Instead of starting with a broad, generalized treatment plan, personalized medicine allows doctors to choose a treatment strategy that's scientifically tailored to the individual's cancer.

The Future of Personalized Medicine

The field of personalized medicine is rapidly evolving, and researchers are continually discovering new genetic mutations, biomarkers, and targeted treatments for breast cancer. As our understanding of cancer's molecular basis grows, doctors will have even more tools to create highly effective and individualized treatment plans.

In the near future, personalized medicine could include **combination therapies**, where multiple treatments are used together to target different aspects of the cancer. There's also a growing focus on **predicting** which treatments will work best for individual patients, minimizing the trial-and-error approach that has been common in cancer treatment.

For patients, this means a future where treatments are not only more effective but also better suited to their personal cancer profile, improving outcomes and enhancing quality of life.

Immunotherapy Breakthroughs

Immunotherapy has emerged as one of the most exciting areas of cancer research in recent years, offering hope for patients with difficult-to-treat cancers, including breast cancer. Unlike traditional treatments such as chemotherapy, which targets both cancer and healthy cells, immunotherapy harnesses the body's own immune system to recognize and destroy cancer cells more specifically. This breakthrough approach has led to remarkable advancements in how we treat breast cancer, particularly for those with aggressive or advanced forms of the disease.

What is Immunotherapy?

Immunotherapy is a type of cancer treatment that works by stimulating the body's immune system to fight cancer more effectively. Normally, the immune system can recognize and destroy abnormal cells, but cancer cells have developed ways to evade detection. Immunotherapy seeks to boost or restore the immune system's ability to identify and attack these cancer cells.

There are several types of immunotherapies, each with its own method of enhancing the immune system's ability to fight cancer. Some of the newer approaches show tremendous promise in the treatment of **breast cancer**, particularly in **triple-negative breast cancer (TNBC)** and **HER2-positive** breast cancer.

New Breakthroughs in Immunotherapy for Breast Cancer

1. Immune Checkpoint Inhibitors

One of the most promising advancements in immunotherapy is the development of **immune checkpoint inhibitors**. These drugs work by blocking certain proteins that prevent the immune system from attacking cancer cells.

- **PD-1 and PD-L1 Inhibitors**: The proteins PD-1 (on immune cells) and PD-L1 (on cancer cells) play a critical role in allowing cancer cells to evade immune detection. Drugs like **pembrolizumab (Keytruda)** and **atezolizumab (Tecentriq)** block these proteins, enabling the immune system to recognize and destroy cancer cells. These inhibitors have shown efficacy in **triple-negative breast cancer (TNBC)**, which is typically harder to treat with standard therapies.

- **CTLA-4 Inhibitors**: **Ipilimumab (Yervoy)** is another checkpoint inhibitor that targets the CTLA-4 protein, which also plays a role in turning off immune responses. When combined with PD-1 inhibitors, these drugs can provide a more robust immune response against cancer cells.

Impact on Breast Cancer: Immunotherapy has been particularly effective for **triple-negative breast cancer**, a subtype that does not express estrogen receptors, progesterone receptors, or HER2. It is typically resistant to hormone therapies and HER2-targeted therapies, making immunotherapy a vital option for these patients.

2. Cancer Vaccines

Cancer vaccines are another exciting frontier in immunotherapy. Unlike traditional vaccines that prevent infections, cancer vaccines aim to stimulate the immune system to target specific cancer cells.

- **Therapeutic Vaccines**: These are designed to treat cancer by teaching the immune system to recognize tumor-specific antigens. One example is **NeuVax**, a vaccine currently being tested for patients with **HER2-positive** breast cancer. The vaccine works by prompting the immune system to attack cells that express the HER2 protein, a key driver of cancer cell growth in many breast cancer patients.

Impact on Breast Cancer: Vaccines like NeuVax hold great promise in preventing recurrence of **HER2-positive** breast cancer and improving long-term outcomes, particularly after surgery or radiation.

3. Adoptive Cell Therapy

Adoptive cell therapy involves taking immune cells from a patient's body, modifying them to better fight cancer, and then reinfusing them into the patient. This innovative approach is still in early stages but has shown potential for cancers that have evaded traditional treatments.

- **CAR T-Cell Therapy**: **Chimeric Antigen Receptor T-cell (CAR-T)** therapy is one of the most advanced forms of adoptive cell therapy. CAR-T cells are genetically engineered to express a receptor specific to cancer cells, allowing the immune system to target and destroy those cells. While CAR-T therapy is currently more commonly used for blood cancers, research is underway to apply it to solid tumors like breast cancer.

Impact on Breast Cancer: Though CAR-T therapy is not yet a standard treatment for breast cancer, it offers hope, especially for aggressive or metastatic breast cancers that do not respond to other treatments.

4. Personalized Cancer Vaccines

In addition to generalized cancer vaccines, there are ongoing efforts to create **personalized vaccines** that are tailored to an individual's tumor. These vaccines would be designed using the patient's unique genetic and molecular tumor profile, enhancing their effectiveness.

- **Neoantigen-based Vaccines**: Neoantigens are unique proteins expressed by cancer cells due to mutations in the tumor's DNA. These vaccines are being developed to target these specific proteins, helping the immune system recognize and destroy the cancer cells.

Impact on Breast Cancer: Neoantigen vaccines could potentially be used to treat **HER2-positive** or **triple-negative** breast cancer, where current treatments are less effective. Personalizing the treatment increases the likelihood of success by targeting the exact genetic changes in the tumor.

5. Combination Immunotherapies

Combining different types of immunotherapy or combining immunotherapy with other treatments such as chemotherapy or targeted therapies is an area of intense research. The goal is to create a more powerful immune response against the tumor by targeting multiple pathways at once.

- **Combination of Checkpoint Inhibitors with Chemotherapy**: For some patients with **triple-negative breast cancer**, combining **chemotherapy** with **checkpoint inhibitors** like pembrolizumab (Keytruda) has resulted in significantly improved outcomes.

- **Combining Immunotherapy with Targeted Therapy**: Another promising approach is combining **HER2-targeted therapies** with immune checkpoint inhibitors. For **HER2-positive** breast cancer, this combination has the potential to enhance the immune system's ability to attack the tumor.

The Future of Immunotherapy in Breast Cancer

As more clinical trials are conducted and new breakthroughs emerge, immunotherapy is becoming an increasingly important tool in the fight against breast cancer. Researchers are continually working to refine these treatments, with the aim of improving their effectiveness and expanding their use to more breast cancer subtypes.

The future of immunotherapy in breast cancer holds the promise of:

- **Better Outcomes for Hard-to-Treat Subtypes**: Immunotherapy is especially valuable for **triple-

negative breast cancer and **HER2-positive** breast cancer, where treatment options were once limited.

- **Longer Survival and Reduced Recurrence**: With advancements in immunotherapy, many patients are living longer, with fewer chances of the cancer coming back.
- **More Personalized Treatment Plans**: As more is learned about the genetic and molecular makeup of breast cancer, immunotherapy treatments will become increasingly personalized, providing the most effective option for each individual.

Targeted Therapies

Targeted therapy is one of the most exciting advances in the treatment of breast cancer. Unlike traditional chemotherapy, which attacks rapidly dividing cells indiscriminately, **targeted therapies** zero in on specific molecules involved in cancer growth, often with greater precision and fewer side effects. These therapies work by blocking the growth and spread of cancer cells by interfering with specific molecules that play a crucial role in the development and progression of breast cancer.

What is Targeted Therapy?

Targeted therapy is designed to target specific molecules or genetic mutations that are involved in the growth and spread of cancer cells. These therapies often work in a way that is different from traditional treatments like chemotherapy or radiation. They can work by:

- **Blocking the signals that cancer cells need to grow**

- **Interfering with the ability of cancer cells to make new blood vessels** (angiogenesis)
- **Delivering toxins or radioactive substances directly to cancer cells**

By focusing on cancer-specific molecular targets, targeted therapies tend to be more effective and less toxic than conventional treatments.

Promising Targeted Therapies for Breast Cancer

1. HER2-Targeted Therapies

One of the most well-known and successful targeted treatments is for **HER2-positive** breast cancer. About **15-20% of breast cancers** overproduce the HER2 protein, which causes the cancer cells to grow and divide uncontrollably. Targeting HER2 has dramatically improved survival rates for patients with this subtype of breast cancer.

- **Trastuzumab (Herceptin)**: One of the earliest and most successful HER2-targeted therapies, **Herceptin** binds to the HER2 protein, blocking the signals that tell the cancer cells to grow. It has been shown to significantly reduce the risk of recurrence and improve survival rates for women with HER2-positive breast cancer.

- **Pertuzumab (Perjeta)**: **Perjeta** works similarly to Herceptin but also targets a different part of the HER2 protein, providing a more powerful effect. When combined with Herceptin and chemotherapy, it has been shown to improve survival outcomes, especially in patients with metastatic HER2-positive breast cancer.

- **Ado-trastuzumab emtansine (Kadcyla)**: This therapy combines **Herceptin** with a chemotherapy drug. It delivers chemotherapy directly to the cancer cells, increasing its effectiveness while minimizing damage to healthy cells. It is often used in patients with metastatic HER2-positive breast cancer who have already been treated with Herceptin.

Impact: These HER2-targeted therapies have transformed the treatment of HER2-positive breast cancer, improving survival rates and quality of life for patients.

2. CDK4/6 Inhibitors for Hormone Receptor-Positive Breast Cancer

Many breast cancers grow in response to **hormones like estrogen and progesterone**, a subtype known as **hormone receptor-positive (HR-positive)** breast cancer. One of the key pathways that allow these cancers to grow is the **CDK4/6 pathway**, which helps cells divide and multiply.

- **Palbociclib (Ibrance)**, **Ribociclib (Kisqali)**, and **Abemaciclib (Verzenio)**: These are **CDK4/6 inhibitors** that target the proteins responsible for driving the growth of HR-positive breast cancer cells. By blocking these proteins, these drugs slow down or stop the cancer cells from dividing.

Impact: CDK4/6 inhibitors have proven to be particularly effective in **advanced or metastatic HR-positive breast cancer**, helping to control tumor growth and prolong life. They are often combined with hormonal therapy to provide a more comprehensive treatment approach.

3. PARP Inhibitors

PARP (Poly ADP-Ribose Polymerase) is an enzyme that helps repair damaged DNA. Cancer cells that have certain genetic mutations, like those in **BRCA1** and **BRCA2**, rely heavily on this repair mechanism to survive. **PARP inhibitors** block this repair process, causing the cancer cells to accumulate DNA damage and eventually die.

- **Olaparib (Lynparza)**: The first **PARP inhibitor** approved for the treatment of breast cancer, **Olaparib** has shown great promise in treating women with **BRCA1 or BRCA2 mutations**, particularly in metastatic or advanced cases.

- **Talazoparib (Talzenna)**: Another PARP inhibitor, **Talazoparib** has also been approved for patients with **germline BRCA mutations**, offering an additional treatment option for those who may not respond to other therapies.

Impact: PARP inhibitors provide an option for patients with **hereditary breast cancers** caused by mutations in the BRCA genes, improving progression-free survival and offering a less toxic alternative to chemotherapy.

4. Angiogenesis Inhibitors

Cancer cells need a blood supply to grow and spread. **Angiogenesis** is the process by which tumors stimulate the formation of new blood vessels. By blocking angiogenesis, these therapies aim to **starve the tumor** by cutting off its blood supply.

- **Bevacizumab (Avastin)**: This angiogenesis inhibitor works by blocking a protein called **VEGF (vascular endothelial growth factor)**, which helps tumors form new blood vessels. Avastin has shown some benefit in certain breast cancer patients, particularly in **metastatic triple-negative breast cancer (TNBC)**.

Impact: While not as widely used as other targeted therapies, angiogenesis inhibitors may provide a treatment option for patients with aggressive or metastatic breast cancers, particularly those that are harder to treat with traditional therapies.

5. T-DM1 (Trastuzumab Emtansine)

This **HER2-targeted therapy** is a combination of the **Herceptin** monoclonal antibody and a chemotherapy drug, which is directly delivered to the cancer cells. **T-DM1** is specifically used for **HER2-positive** metastatic breast cancer after other treatments, such as trastuzumab (Herceptin) or chemotherapy, have failed.

Impact: T-DM1 has been shown to improve survival and reduce side effects by delivering chemotherapy directly to the cancer cells while minimizing damage to healthy tissue.

6. Immuno-Targeted Therapies: Combining Immunotherapy with Targeted Treatment

Some of the **newer immunotherapies** are being combined with targeted therapies to enhance effectiveness. For example, **HER2-targeted therapies** like **Trastuzumab** are being paired with **immune checkpoint inhibitors** (like **Pembrolizumab**) to improve outcomes for patients with **HER2-positive breast cancer**. This combination aims to not only target the cancer but also boost the immune system's ability to fight the tumor.

The Future of Targeted Therapies

Targeted therapies are constantly evolving, and new drug combinations, delivery methods, and treatment regimens are continually being developed. In the future, we can expect to see:

- **More specific and personalized treatments**, with therapies tailored to the individual's genetic and molecular profile.
- **Fewer side effects** and more effective treatment options, as drugs become more targeted and less toxic.

- **Combination therapies** that pair targeted therapies with immunotherapies, chemotherapy, or radiation, improving efficacy for hard-to-treat cancers.

Early Detection Innovations

Early detection of breast cancer is key to improving survival rates, as finding the cancer in its earliest stages often means more effective treatment options and a higher chance of successful outcomes. While traditional methods like mammograms and ultrasounds remain essential, **innovative screening techniques** are emerging to improve early detection, especially for hard-to-diagnose cases. Among the most exciting breakthroughs is the development of **liquid biopsies**, a less invasive method that analyzes cancer-related DNA found in the blood.

What are Liquid Biopsies?

A **liquid biopsy** is a cutting-edge screening tool that detects cancer-related changes in a person's blood, primarily by identifying fragments of **circulating tumor DNA (ctDNA)**, which are bits of genetic material shed by cancer cells into the bloodstream. Unlike traditional biopsies that involve taking tissue samples directly from the tumor, liquid biopsies use a simple blood draw to assess cancer-related biomarkers, offering a much less invasive approach.

This technique has the potential to detect cancer at very **early stages**, sometimes even before a tumor is visible through imaging techniques like mammograms. Liquid biopsies can also be used to monitor the **progression of cancer** or detect **recurrence** after treatment.

How Liquid Biopsies Work

Liquid biopsies work by detecting and analyzing **circulating tumor DNA (ctDNA)** or **circulating tumor cells (CTCs)** found in a patient's blood. Here's a simplified breakdown of how the process works:

1. **Blood Draw**: A blood sample is taken, usually from the arm.
2. **DNA Extraction**: The blood is processed to separate out the plasma, and the DNA is extracted from the plasma.
3. **Analysis**: Specialized tests analyze the genetic material for mutations, alterations, or markers associated with cancer. These markers may indicate the presence of a tumor, even if it's too small to detect through other methods.
4. **Interpretation**: Doctors use the results to understand whether cancer is present, assess the tumor's genetic makeup, and guide treatment decisions.

Unlike traditional biopsies, liquid biopsies are **non-invasive**, can be performed more frequently, and **don't carry the risk** of complications like infections or bleeding, making them a promising option for regular monitoring.

The Benefits of Liquid Biopsies for Early Detection

1. Early Detection of Breast Cancer

One of the biggest advantages of liquid biopsies is their ability to detect cancer at very **early stages**. Because ctDNA is shed into the bloodstream by even the smallest of tumors, liquid biopsies could potentially identify **breast cancer years before it is visible on a mammogram or ultrasound**. This could mean that patients could start treatment much earlier, giving them a better chance of recovery and a less aggressive treatment plan.

In fact, some early research suggests that liquid biopsies may even be able to detect **microscopic cancer cells** that may not yet form a palpable lump, offering a new approach to cancer screening that's more **sensitive** and **precise** than traditional imaging methods.

2. Monitoring Treatment Response

Liquid biopsies are not only useful for initial detection but also for **monitoring treatment response**. During cancer treatment, patients may undergo multiple rounds of chemotherapy, radiation, or targeted therapies. Liquid biopsies can be used to see if the cancer is **shrinking** or if the therapy is having an impact on the ctDNA levels in the blood.

Additionally, liquid biopsies can help detect **minimal residual disease**—tiny cancerous cells that remain in the body after treatment, which could eventually lead to recurrence. By detecting these small traces of cancer DNA, doctors can make adjustments to the treatment plan before the cancer has a chance to regrow.

3. Detecting Cancer Recurrence

For patients in remission, one of the biggest concerns is whether the cancer will return. Liquid biopsies can be used to detect even the smallest traces of cancer cells in the bloodstream long before they show up on other tests like mammograms. This allows doctors to **catch recurrences early**, often while they are still localized and easier to treat.

A major advantage is that liquid biopsies allow for regular, non-invasive monitoring. This means doctors can perform tests more frequently without the discomfort or risks associated with repeated traditional biopsies or imaging.

Other Innovations in Early Detection

While liquid biopsies are among the most exciting innovations in early detection, other advances are also being made to improve breast cancer screening:

1. Artificial Intelligence (AI) in Mammography

AI is being integrated into mammography to improve the accuracy of screening and reduce human error. By analyzing mammogram images, AI systems can detect abnormalities that might be missed by human eyes, potentially leading to earlier diagnosis and more accurate assessments.

2. Molecular Breast Imaging (MBI)

Molecular breast imaging uses a special radiotracer to identify areas of high metabolic activity, a hallmark of cancer. This imaging technique is especially useful in women with dense breast tissue, where traditional mammograms can miss tumors.

3. 3D Mammography (Tomosynthesis)

3D mammography, also known as **tomosynthesis**, provides a more detailed image of the breast by taking multiple X-ray images from different angles. This allows for better visualization of dense breast tissue and can reduce the number of false positives, leading to fewer unnecessary biopsies.

Challenges and Limitations of Liquid Biopsies

Although liquid biopsies are a major breakthrough, they are not without limitations:

- **Detection Sensitivity**: While liquid biopsies are promising, they are still being perfected for early-stage detection. In some cases, particularly with smaller tumors, ctDNA may not be present in detectable amounts, potentially leading to **false negatives**.

- **Cost and Accessibility**: As with any new technology, liquid biopsies are currently expensive, and not all healthcare systems have access to the necessary tools or resources for testing.

- **Lack of Standardization**: Since liquid biopsy tests are still relatively new, there is a need for **standardized protocols** and further validation to ensure they are reliable and accurate for widespread clinical use.

The Future of Early Detection

Despite the current challenges, **liquid biopsies** and other **innovative screening methods** represent a promising future for breast cancer detection. Researchers are optimistic that with continued advancements in technology, these techniques will become more sensitive, affordable, and widely accessible, leading to **earlier, more accurate diagnoses**. For now, they offer hope for a less invasive, more precise way to detect and monitor breast cancer, empowering patients and doctors alike to stay ahead of the disease.

As liquid biopsy technology improves, it's possible that one day, a simple blood test could become part of the routine screening process for all women, revolutionizing breast cancer care and potentially saving countless lives by detecting the disease at its earliest, most treatable stages.

Preventive Treatments

For individuals at high risk of developing breast cancer, the idea of preventing the disease before it begins is both a hopeful and crucial part of the conversation. While regular screenings are essential for early detection, **preventive treatments**—also known as **chemoprevention**—are another powerful strategy in the fight against breast cancer. Medications like **Tamoxifen** have been proven to reduce the risk of breast cancer in high-risk individuals, and researchers continue to explore new alternatives that may be even more effective or have fewer side effects.

What is Chemoprevention?

Chemoprevention refers to the use of specific drugs, vitamins, or other substances to try to **lower the risk of cancer**. For breast cancer, chemoprevention is typically recommended for individuals at **high risk** due to factors like family history, genetic mutations (such as BRCA1 or BRCA2), or other inherited conditions that increase the likelihood of developing breast cancer. Rather than treating cancer once it appears, chemoprevention aims to **prevent the disease from occurring in the first place** or to slow its progression in those who may already have precancerous changes in their cells.

Tamoxifen: A Well-Known Preventive Treatment

Tamoxifen is one of the most well-known and widely prescribed drugs for preventing breast cancer, particularly in women who are at a **higher risk**. It is a **selective estrogen receptor modulator (SERM)**, which means it works by interfering with the action of estrogen—a hormone that can fuel the growth of certain types of breast cancer.

How Tamoxifen Works

Tamoxifen blocks estrogen from binding to estrogen receptors on the surface of breast cancer cells, **slowing their growth**. In high-risk women, particularly those with a family history of breast cancer or those carrying the **BRCA mutations**, Tamoxifen can lower the risk of developing estrogen-receptor-positive breast cancers. It is typically used in women who are either **pre-menopausal** or **post-menopausal**, although it is generally more effective in pre-menopausal women.

Tamoxifen has been shown to reduce the risk of developing **breast cancer by 30-50%** in high-risk women and is typically taken for **5 years** as a preventive measure. It is also used in the treatment of estrogen receptor-positive breast cancers.

Alternatives to Tamoxifen

While Tamoxifen is an effective preventive treatment, some individuals may not be able to tolerate it due to side effects, or they may require alternatives. Fortunately, there are several other medications that work in similar ways to Tamoxifen and may offer **different benefits** or fewer risks.

1. Raloxifene

Raloxifene is another **SERM** that is sometimes used for breast cancer prevention, particularly in post-menopausal women. Like Tamoxifen, it works by blocking estrogen receptors on breast cells, but it also has a slightly different profile when it comes to side effects.

- **How it works**: Raloxifene blocks estrogen receptors in breast tissue but may have less of an effect on other tissues (like the uterus), which can reduce some of the side effects seen with Tamoxifen, such as the risk of uterine cancer.

- **Effectiveness**: Studies show that Raloxifene can reduce breast cancer risk by approximately **38%** in postmenopausal women who are at high risk, similar to Tamoxifen.

- **Side effects**: While it may have a more favorable side effect profile in some women, Raloxifene still carries some risks, including an increased chance of **blood clots** and **stroke**.

2. Aromatase Inhibitors

Aromatase inhibitors, such as **Anastrozole**, **Letrozole**, and **Exemestane**, are medications that reduce the amount of estrogen in the body by inhibiting the enzyme **aromatase**, which converts other hormones into estrogen. These drugs are commonly used to treat breast cancer in postmenopausal women, but they are also being studied as preventive treatments.

- **How they work**: By reducing estrogen levels, aromatase inhibitors lower the stimulation of estrogen receptor-positive cancer cells.

- **Effectiveness**: Studies suggest that aromatase inhibitors can reduce breast cancer risk in postmenopausal women by up to **50%**, and they are typically more effective than Tamoxifen for women who are already postmenopausal.

- **Side effects**: Common side effects of aromatase inhibitors include **joint pain**, **hot flashes**, and an increased risk of **osteoporosis** due to the lowering of estrogen levels.

These medications are often considered for women who are at high risk and have already completed menopause, as they are generally **less effective in pre-menopausal women**.

3. Exemestane (Aromasin)

Exemestane is another aromatase inhibitor that has been studied for breast cancer prevention, particularly in postmenopausal women at high risk. In some studies, it has been found to be more effective than Tamoxifen for preventing hormone receptor-positive breast cancer in postmenopausal women.

- **Effectiveness**: Exemestane has been shown to reduce the risk of developing breast cancer by up to **65%** in high-risk women, though it is more commonly used in women who have already been diagnosed with breast cancer as part of adjuvant therapy.

Choosing the Right Preventive Treatment

When deciding on a preventive treatment plan, doctors will take into account several factors, including:

- **Personal risk level**: A woman's genetic makeup, family history, and other health factors will influence the decision.
- **Menopausal status**: Postmenopausal women may benefit more from aromatase inhibitors, while premenopausal women may be prescribed Tamoxifen or Raloxifene.
- **Side effect profiles**: Each medication comes with its own set of potential side effects. For instance, some women may not tolerate the side effects of Tamoxifen and may prefer an alternative like Raloxifene or aromatase inhibitors.

Ultimately, it's important for individuals to discuss their options thoroughly with their healthcare team. Chemoprevention can be a powerful tool for high-risk individuals, but each patient's personal preferences, risk factors, and medical history must be considered to find the most suitable treatment.

The Future of Preventive Treatments

The field of breast cancer prevention continues to evolve, with researchers looking for new and **better ways to prevent** the disease. In addition to the medications mentioned above, **clinical trials** are ongoing to test new preventive treatments, including drugs that target specific genes or pathways involved in cancer development. Some new medications aim to **block cancer cell growth more effectively** while reducing the side effects associated with traditional treatments like Tamoxifen.

Chapter 10: Living with Breast Cancer

Survivorship

Survivorship, when it comes to breast cancer, means more than just the absence of disease. It's about reclaiming your life after treatment, navigating the challenges of recovery, and embracing the possibility of a future filled with new opportunities and experiences. Being a **breast cancer survivor** means you've undergone treatment, emerged on the other side, and are now focused on moving forward. But what does that journey look like? And what does it truly mean to be a **survivor**?

What Does It Mean to Be a Breast Cancer Survivor?

The definition of a **cancer survivor** can differ from person to person, but it generally refers to anyone who has been diagnosed with cancer and has completed their primary treatment. In the case of breast cancer, survivorship begins the moment active treatment ends, whether that's surgery, chemotherapy, radiation, or a combination.

The **National Cancer Institute** defines a survivor as anyone who has been diagnosed with cancer, from the moment of diagnosis through the balance of their life. **Breast cancer survivors** include those who are **cancer-free** as well as those living with the disease as a chronic condition.

Survivorship isn't just about being free of cancer—it's about **navigating the complexities of life after treatment**. Survivors often face unique challenges, both physically and emotionally, and they must find ways to manage these challenges while continuing to live fulfilling, healthy lives.

Long-Term Effects of Breast Cancer Treatment

While many breast cancer survivors live long, healthy lives post-treatment, it's important to understand that the journey doesn't end when treatment finishes. Survivors may experience both **physical and emotional long-term effects** that require attention and care. These can include:

1. Physical Effects

- **Fatigue**: Fatigue is a common long-term effect, especially after chemotherapy and radiation. It can persist for months or even years after treatment. It's important to address this with **rest**, a balanced diet, and **gentle exercise**.

- **Lymphedema**: This condition occurs when the lymph nodes are damaged or removed, often during surgery. It can cause swelling in the arm or chest area, which may require physical therapy or the use of compression garments.

- **Bone Health**: Some treatments, particularly chemotherapy and hormone therapy, can impact **bone density**, increasing the risk of **osteoporosis**. Survivors are encouraged to engage in weight-bearing exercises, eat calcium-rich foods, and discuss **bone health** with their healthcare providers.

- **Menopause**: For some women, chemotherapy or hormone therapy can cause **early menopause**. This can lead to symptoms like hot flashes, vaginal dryness, and mood changes, which may require medical management.

- **Heart Health**: Certain breast cancer treatments, such as **chemotherapy** and **radiation therapy**, may increase the risk of heart issues later in life. Regular checkups and monitoring are important to detect any potential complications early.

2. Emotional and Psychological Effects

- **Anxiety and Fear of Recurrence**: One of the most common challenges after treatment is the constant worry that cancer could return. Survivors may experience **anxiety**, depression, or emotional stress, often referred to as **survivorship stress**. Learning to manage this fear with the help of therapy or support groups can be vital for mental well-being.

- **Body Image Concerns**: Breast cancer treatment often involves surgery (e.g., mastectomy or lumpectomy), and many women may struggle with body image issues after losing a breast or going through significant physical changes. This is normal, and there are many options available for emotional support, including **reconstruction surgery**, **prosthetics**, and **counseling**.

- **Mental Health**: Emotional well-being is just as important as physical health. Survivors might experience feelings of **depression, isolation**, or **anger**. It's important for survivors to seek help from **mental health professionals** or **support groups** to navigate these emotions.

Living a Fulfilling Life Post-Treatment

Breast cancer survivorship is not just about surviving—it's about thriving. After the treatment phase ends, it's time to focus on **living life fully** again. Many survivors go on to lead fulfilling lives, embracing the opportunities that come with a new perspective on health and life. Here are some ways to live well after treatment:

1. Prioritize Health and Wellness

- **Nutrition**: Eating a healthy, well-balanced diet is crucial for maintaining energy and managing long-term effects. Focusing on **whole foods, fruits and vegetables**, lean proteins, and **healthy fats** can provide the nutrients needed for ongoing recovery and overall well-being.

- **Exercise**: Moderate physical activity can greatly improve energy levels, reduce the risk of recurrence, and help manage anxiety or depression. Survivors should aim for **regular exercise**, such as walking, swimming, or yoga, as well as strength-building exercises for bone health.

- **Regular Check-Ups**: After treatment, survivors will continue with **regular check-ups** to monitor for any signs of recurrence and manage ongoing health concerns. These may include physical exams, mammograms, blood tests, and other screenings. Staying consistent with follow-up appointments is essential.

2. Manage Emotional Well-Being

- **Support Networks**: Family, friends, and **support groups** play a huge role in recovery. Emotional support from loved ones can help survivors navigate difficult moments and maintain a sense of connection. Support groups, whether in person or online, offer the opportunity to share experiences with others who understand what it's like to live through cancer treatment and recovery.

- **Mental Health Support**: Therapy, mindfulness, and **meditation** techniques can help survivors manage anxiety, depression, and stress. Cognitive behavioral therapy (CBT) is often recommended to help individuals reframe negative thought patterns and focus on positive aspects of life.

- **Mindfulness Practices**: Incorporating practices such as **meditation**, **deep breathing**, and **mindfulness** can help reduce the impact of stress and enhance emotional resilience.

3. Find Meaning and Purpose

- **Embrace New Beginnings**: Survivorship often comes with a newfound appreciation for life. Many survivors decide to **pursue new passions**, whether it's taking up a hobby, starting a new career, or traveling. Cancer can offer an opportunity to reflect on what truly matters, and some survivors use this time to **advocate** for breast cancer awareness or help others going through similar experiences.

- **Focus on Relationships**: Cancer can alter relationships, and survivors often find that their connections with loved ones deepen after treatment. This is a time to **reconnect** with family and friends, nurturing relationships that matter most.

4. Celebrate Milestones

- **Survivorship Anniversaries**: Many survivors celebrate the **anniversary of their diagnosis** or the completion of their treatment. These milestones can be marked with personal reflections, community events, or simply spending time with loved ones.

- **Living in the Moment**: Taking the time to appreciate the small moments in life—whether it's a quiet morning with a cup of coffee, time spent with family, or achieving a personal goal—can help survivors focus on the present and enjoy life after treatment.

Long-Term Follow-Up

After completing treatment for breast cancer, the journey doesn't end. **Long-term follow-up** is crucial in ensuring that any potential recurrence or new health concerns are caught early, offering the best chance for successful intervention. Regular monitoring and check-ups are not only important for detecting a recurrence but also for managing long-term effects of treatment and maintaining overall health.

Why Long-Term Follow-Up is Necessary

While the end of active treatment often brings a sense of relief, the fear of **cancer recurrence** is very real for many survivors. In fact, breast cancer can come back months or even years after treatment. This is why **follow-up care** is essential. It allows healthcare providers to closely monitor your health, identify any changes in your body, and catch any signs of recurrence as early as possible, when treatment is most effective.

Regular check-ups help detect the following:

- **Local Recurrence**: This refers to the cancer returning in the same area where it started, such as the breast or chest wall.

- **Distant Recurrence**: Sometimes, cancer cells spread to other parts of the body (like bones, liver, or lungs). Detecting this early through tests and imaging can improve treatment options.

- **Late Side Effects of Treatment**: Long-term follow-up also includes managing the side effects of cancer treatments that may develop over time, such as heart problems, lymphedema, or osteoporosis.

What Does Long-Term Follow-Up Involve?

Long-term follow-up usually begins after a survivor has completed their primary cancer treatment and is in **remission** (no visible signs of cancer). The follow-up process will vary depending on the type of breast cancer, the treatments used, and individual health needs, but generally includes the following elements:

1. Regular Physical Exams

Your healthcare provider will conduct **regular physical exams**, which may involve checking for any physical signs of recurrence, such as:

- **Changes in the breast or chest area** (new lumps, changes in size, skin changes)
- **Changes in the lymph nodes** (swelling, firmness, or tenderness)
- **General health checks** to monitor the impact of past treatments.

These exams are typically scheduled every **3-6 months** during the first 3 years after treatment, and then once a year thereafter, depending on the doctor's recommendation.

2. Imaging Tests

Imaging tests like **mammograms**, **ultrasounds**, and **MRIs** play a key role in identifying any signs of recurrence or other health issues.

- **Mammograms** are the primary imaging tool used for monitoring breast health. They are usually performed once a year, but your doctor may recommend them more frequently if you have a higher risk of recurrence.

- **Breast MRI** may be used in certain situations, such as for women with dense breasts or high-risk patients.
- **Ultrasounds** may be performed if there is a specific concern or lump to examine in more detail.

3. Blood Tests

While there is no routine blood test to detect breast cancer recurrence, doctors may order **blood tests** to check for changes that might indicate a recurrence or the presence of cancer in other parts of the body. For instance, **tumor markers** may be tested in certain cases to help monitor for recurrence.

4. Bone Density Tests

Certain treatments for breast cancer, such as chemotherapy and hormone therapy, can weaken bones over time. **Bone density tests** (DEXA scans) are often recommended for survivors who received these treatments to check for signs of **osteoporosis**.

5. Heart Health Monitoring

If you received certain treatments like **chemotherapy** (especially anthracyclines) or **radiation therapy**, regular monitoring of heart health may be necessary, as these treatments can have long-term effects on heart function. Tests like **echocardiograms** or **EKGs** may be recommended to ensure your heart is functioning properly.

How Often Should You Have Follow-Up Visits?

The frequency of follow-up visits will depend on the individual's health, risk factors, and the type of breast cancer they had. In general, follow-up appointments are scheduled as follows:

- **Years 1-3**: Every **3-6 months** for the first 3 years.
- **Years 4-5**: Every **6-12 months**.
- **Year 6 and beyond**: Annually or as needed, depending on health and risk factors.

Follow-up care will evolve over time, and the intensity of monitoring may decrease if no recurrence is detected in the earlier years.

The Importance of Self-Advocacy

While your healthcare team plays an essential role in monitoring your health, it's also important for you to **advocate for yourself**. If you notice any changes in your body, no matter how small or seemingly insignificant, it's vital to bring them to your doctor's attention immediately. Early detection of recurrence significantly improves the chances of successful treatment and can provide you with peace of mind.

What to Expect Emotionally During Follow-Up Care

For many survivors, the emotional journey continues long after treatment ends. The fear of recurrence can be overwhelming, and regular check-ups may trigger **anxiety** or **stress**. It's important to acknowledge these feelings and seek support when needed. **Therapy**, **support groups**, and **mindfulness techniques** can be beneficial for managing the emotional toll of regular check-ups and the uncertainty of the future.

Quality of Life

Breast cancer treatment can take a significant toll on both the body and mind, and the journey to recovery can be challenging. But it's important to remember that **quality of life** matters just as much as survival. Life after treatment often involves adjusting to a new reality, navigating changes in your physical and emotional health, and finding ways to thrive in your daily life.

Managing Fatigue: A Common Aftereffect

Fatigue is one of the most common and persistent side effects of breast cancer treatment. It can linger long after chemotherapy and radiation have ended. It's important to recognize that this fatigue is different from ordinary tiredness, and pushing through it can actually make it worse.

Practical Tips:

- **Prioritize Rest:** Take short naps when needed, but try to avoid long periods of inactivity during the day, as it may worsen fatigue.

- **Pace Yourself:** Break up tasks into smaller steps and rest in between. Don't feel pressure to do everything in one go.

- **Stay Active:** Light exercise can actually help reduce fatigue in the long run. Walking, swimming, or yoga can boost energy levels and improve overall health. Start slow, and listen to your body.

- **Stay Hydrated:** Drink plenty of water and eat nutrient-rich foods to fuel your body and avoid dehydration, which can worsen fatigue.

Improving Sleep: Combatting Insomnia

Many survivors struggle with **insomnia** or disrupted sleep patterns following breast cancer treatment. This may be due to hormonal changes, the stress of the diagnosis, or physical discomfort.

Practical Tips:

- **Create a Sleep Routine:** Try to go to bed and wake up at the same time each day, even on weekends. A consistent sleep schedule helps reset your body's internal clock.

- **Create a Relaxing Sleep Environment:** Keep your bedroom cool, dark, and quiet. Consider using blackout curtains or an eye mask, and try white noise machines or earplugs if noise is an issue.

- **Limit Stimulants:** Avoid caffeine, nicotine, or alcohol close to bedtime, as they can disrupt sleep. Instead, opt for herbal teas like chamomile or valerian root, which promote relaxation.

- **Mindfulness & Relaxation Techniques:** Practices like deep breathing, progressive muscle relaxation, or meditation can calm the mind and prepare you for a restful night's sleep.

Nurturing Relationships: Connecting with Loved Ones

Going through breast cancer treatment can put a strain on relationships. Partners, family members, and friends may struggle to understand what you're going through, and you may feel emotionally distant or overwhelmed.

Practical Tips:

- **Communicate Openly:** Be honest about your needs and feelings. Let your loved ones know what kind of support you need, whether it's physical help, emotional support, or just someone to talk to.

- **Set Boundaries:** It's okay to ask for alone time when needed. Let people know when you're feeling overwhelmed or need space to rest.

- **Lean on Support Groups:** Sometimes, the people closest to you may not fully understand the emotional or physical toll of breast cancer. Connecting with others in similar situations can provide a sense of community and reduce feelings of isolation.

- **Seek Couples Counseling:** If your relationship has been strained, consider therapy to work through emotional difficulties and rediscover connection with your partner.

Managing Stress and Anxiety: Coping with the Emotional Impact

Living with the uncertainty of recurrence or adjusting to life after cancer can cause significant **stress** and **anxiety**. Managing these emotions is essential for improving your mental well-being and overall quality of life.

Practical Tips:

- **Mindfulness and Meditation:** Mindfulness practices can help you stay present and reduce anxiety. Start with 5-10 minutes of deep breathing or guided meditation each day.

- **Journaling:** Writing about your thoughts and emotions can be a therapeutic way to process what you've been through and what you're feeling now.

- **Therapy or Counseling:** Seeing a therapist or counselor who specializes in cancer-related emotional support can be incredibly helpful. Cognitive Behavioral Therapy (CBT) can help you manage negative thoughts and stress.

- **Practice Self-Compassion:** It's normal to feel a range of emotions after cancer treatment. Be gentle with yourself and allow yourself to feel your feelings without judgment.

Nutrition and Hydration: Fueling Your Body for Wellness

Maintaining a **healthy diet** is essential for physical recovery and overall health. Many survivors face challenges with appetite, digestion, or maintaining a balanced diet during or after treatment, but the right foods can help promote healing, manage side effects, and boost energy levels.

Practical Tips:

- **Eat Nutrient-Rich Foods:** Focus on whole, unprocessed foods, including fruits, vegetables, lean proteins, whole grains, and healthy fats. These provide vital nutrients to support your recovery.

- **Consider Small Meals:** If you have trouble eating large meals, try eating smaller, more frequent meals throughout the day to keep your energy up.

- **Manage Side Effects:** If you're experiencing nausea, try ginger or peppermint tea. If you're dealing with a loss of appetite, opt for calorie-dense, nutritious snacks, like smoothies or nuts.

- **Hydrate:** Drink plenty of water to stay hydrated, especially if you're experiencing dryness or dehydration from medications.

Staying Active: Improving Physical and Mental Health

Exercise isn't just good for your body—it's beneficial for your mind, too. Even moderate activity can improve mood, reduce stress, and increase energy levels during recovery.

Practical Tips:

- **Start Slowly:** If you've been inactive for a while, begin with gentle activities like walking, yoga, or stretching. Gradually increase the intensity as your strength returns.
- **Exercise with a Friend:** If motivation is a challenge, ask a friend or family member to join you for walks or light exercise. Socializing while being active can help you stay committed.
- **Find Joy in Movement:** Try different forms of exercise, like dancing or swimming, to find what you enjoy most. The goal is to make movement a fun part of your routine.

Finding Purpose: Embracing New Hobbies and Goals

Living through breast cancer may lead to a reassessment of your life and priorities. Many survivors find new purpose through hobbies, volunteering, or pursuing personal goals after treatment.

Practical Tips:

- **Explore New Interests:** Take up a hobby you've always wanted to try, whether it's painting, writing, gardening, or learning a new language. Doing something you enjoy can improve your overall sense of well-being.

- **Set New Goals:** Focus on what you want to achieve in the next chapter of your life, whether it's personal, professional, or emotional growth. Setting small, achievable goals can help you feel accomplished and motivated.
- **Volunteer:** Giving back to others can provide a sense of purpose. Consider volunteering at a cancer support organization or other community-based activities.

Managing Financial Stress: Taking Control of Your Finances

Dealing with the financial burden of cancer treatment can be overwhelming. After treatment, it's important to address any lingering financial worries.

Practical Tips:

- **Review Insurance and Coverage:** Make sure your insurance is up to date and covers any follow-up care or medications you may need. Reach out to a financial advisor if you're unsure of your options.
- **Seek Financial Support:** Many cancer organizations offer financial assistance for survivors who need help covering costs related to follow-up care, medication, or even day-to-day living expenses.

Seeking Financial Support

After the active treatment phase of breast cancer, survivors may still face financial burdens related to follow-up care, medications, and the general costs of daily living. Fortunately, many organizations offer financial assistance programs designed to support cancer survivors in these areas.

Cancer-Specific Financial Assistance Programs

Several organizations offer direct financial aid to cancer survivors to help them manage the costs of their ongoing care. These programs are often aimed at covering medical expenses, follow-up treatments, and medications that may not be fully covered by insurance.

Notable Programs:

- **The American Cancer Society (ACS):** The ACS provides financial support to cancer patients and survivors through grants, co-pay assistance, and transportation support. They also offer resources on managing healthcare costs and connecting survivors with financial counselors.

- **CancerCare:** This organization offers financial assistance for cancer survivors to help with co-pays for medications, transportation costs, and other cancer-related expenses. They also provide free counseling and support services.

- **The Pink Fund:** This nonprofit organization provides short-term financial aid for breast cancer patients and survivors who are in active treatment or recovering. It covers living expenses such as rent, utilities, and health insurance premiums.

Medication Assistance Programs

Cancer survivors often need ongoing medication for hormone therapy, targeted therapies, or managing side effects. These medications can be expensive, and insurance may not always cover the full cost.

Resources:

- **Patient Assistance Programs (PAPs):** Many pharmaceutical companies have programs that provide medications at reduced or no cost for qualified patients. These programs are typically available for brand-name medications, including cancer treatments.
- **NeedyMeds:** This website helps cancer survivors find assistance programs for medications and other health-related expenses. They offer a searchable database for patient assistance programs, discounts, and free health services.
- **GoodRx:** This service allows patients to compare medication prices at different pharmacies and find coupons to reduce out-of-pocket costs.

Transportation and Housing Assistance

Cancer treatment can require frequent visits to medical facilities, which can lead to significant transportation costs, especially for survivors who live far from treatment centers. Additionally, housing costs may increase if survivors need to relocate temporarily for treatment or follow-up care.

Support Options:

- **The American Cancer Society (ACS) Road to Recovery Program:** This program offers free transportation services to and from cancer treatment appointments for individuals who cannot drive or afford transportation.
- **The Leukemia & Lymphoma Society (LLS):** While focused on blood cancers, LLS offers transportation support for cancer patients, including help with fuel and rides to medical appointments.

- **National Cancer Institute (NCI):** NCI offers links to resources for survivors, including programs that provide assistance with lodging and travel costs for treatment.

Utility and Living Expense Assistance

For many cancer survivors, ongoing treatment and follow-up care can result in time off work, leading to a reduction in income. Several organizations provide support to help cover the cost of utilities, rent, and other essential living expenses.

Programs to Explore:

- **The HealthWell Foundation:** The HealthWell Foundation provides financial assistance for cancer patients and survivors to help with health insurance premiums, co-pays, and other out-of-pocket medical costs.

- **The United Way:** Some local United Way chapters offer assistance with utility bills, rent, and groceries for individuals in need, including cancer survivors. These services are often available on a case-by-case basis.

- **Salvation Army and Catholic Charities:** These organizations provide emergency financial assistance for housing, food, and utilities. Many local branches offer grants or direct financial help for individuals facing financial hardship due to health-related issues.

Crowdfunding and Community Support

In addition to formal financial assistance programs, crowdfunding platforms and community support can be valuable resources for cancer survivors. These platforms allow individuals to raise money for medical expenses, treatment costs, and day-to-day living needs.

Options to Consider:

- **GoFundMe:** A popular crowdfunding platform that allows cancer survivors to create fundraising pages to help cover medical bills, transportation costs, and other expenses. Support from friends, family, and even strangers can provide a significant financial cushion.

- **Fundraising Events:** Some communities and local organizations host fundraising events, such as charity runs or auctions, to help cancer survivors pay for ongoing medical needs. Consider reaching out to local cancer support groups or organizations for information on upcoming events.

Financial Counseling and Planning Services

Understanding how to manage finances during and after cancer treatment can be overwhelming. Several organizations offer financial counseling services to help cancer survivors navigate the complexities of managing costs, budgeting, and planning for the future.

Resources Available:

- **Cancer and Careers:** This nonprofit organization offers resources for cancer survivors returning to work, including information about workplace rights, job accommodations, and career planning. They also provide advice on managing finances during treatment.

- **Cancer Financial Assistance Coalition (CFAC):** This coalition is a group of organizations that provide free resources for cancer patients and survivors, including financial assistance, planning tips, and information on available financial aid programs.

Government Programs

Survivors who are experiencing financial difficulty may also be eligible for government assistance programs such as food stamps (SNAP), temporary assistance for needy families (TANF), and Medicaid.

Eligibility Requirements:

- **Medicaid:** Medicaid is a government-funded health insurance program for low-income individuals, including cancer survivors. Depending on income and eligibility, survivors may be able to receive coverage for follow-up care, medication, and treatment-related expenses.

- **Supplemental Nutrition Assistance Program (SNAP):** Cancer survivors who are struggling to pay for food may be eligible for SNAP benefits, which provide financial assistance for groceries.

- **Social Security Disability Insurance (SSDI):** If a cancer survivor is unable to return to work due to long-term effects of treatment or illness, they may qualify for SSDI benefits.

Tax Relief

Cancer survivors may be eligible for tax deductions or credits to help reduce the financial strain. Some of these benefits can help offset medical expenses or provide relief if a survivor is unable to work.

Options for Consideration:

- **Medical Expense Deduction:** As mentioned earlier, the IRS allows individuals to deduct medical expenses that exceed a certain percentage of their income. This can include costs associated with treatment, travel for medical visits, and prescription medications.

- **Earned Income Tax Credit (EITC):** If a survivor's income is significantly reduced due to their diagnosis and they meet the requirements, they may qualify for the EITC, which can provide a significant tax refund.

Legal and Financial Considerations

A breast cancer diagnosis doesn't just affect your health—it can also have significant financial and legal implications. The costs of treatment, potential time off work, and changes in insurance coverage can create financial stress, while there may also be legal concerns to address, such as your rights in the workplace or estate planning.

Understanding these factors and planning ahead can help ease the burden during a difficult time. Below are some key areas to consider:

Health Insurance and Coverage: Understanding Your Options

Breast cancer treatment can be expensive, and navigating insurance coverage is a critical aspect of managing the financial impact. Whether you have private insurance, employer-provided insurance, or government assistance, understanding your benefits and potential out-of-pocket costs is essential.

Practical Tips:

- **Review Your Coverage:** Contact your insurance provider to understand what is covered under your plan. Ensure that your treatments, medications, doctor visits, and any hospital stays are covered. Be clear about which services might require prior authorization.

- **Out-of-Pocket Costs:** Be aware of co-pays, deductibles, and out-of-pocket maximums. Ask your insurance company for an estimate of what you'll pay for treatments, medications, and other care.

- **Financial Assistance Programs:** Many pharmaceutical companies, hospitals, and non-profit organizations offer assistance programs to help cover the cost of medications and treatments. Don't hesitate to reach out and inquire about these programs.

- **Appealing Denied Claims:** If your insurance denies coverage for a treatment or service, know that you have the right to appeal. Many insurers have a formal appeals process, and it's worth pursuing, especially if your doctor supports the treatment.

Disability and Employment Rights: Knowing Your Legal Rights in the Workplace

A cancer diagnosis may impact your ability to work, but there are legal protections in place to help you navigate this. Understanding your rights in the workplace is essential to ensure you are not penalized or discriminated against because of your health condition.

Practical Tips:

- **Family and Medical Leave Act (FMLA):** In the U.S., the FMLA allows eligible employees to take up to 12 weeks of unpaid leave per year for medical reasons, including cancer treatment. This time off is job-protected, meaning your employer cannot fire you for taking leave. However, FMLA only applies to employees who work for covered employers and meet certain eligibility criteria.

- **Americans with Disabilities Act (ADA):** If your cancer diagnosis qualifies as a disability, you may be protected by the ADA. This law prohibits discrimination based on disability and requires employers to provide reasonable accommodations, such as flexible working hours or modified duties, to help you continue working during treatment.

- **Short-Term Disability Insurance:** If you have short-term disability insurance, it may provide income replacement while you're unable to work due to your diagnosis or treatment. Be sure to check the terms of your policy to understand what is covered and how long benefits last.

- **Long-Term Disability Insurance:** If your condition will prevent you from working for an extended period, long-term disability insurance can provide more long-term financial support. This coverage typically begins after short-term disability benefits end and may continue until you can return to work or reach retirement age.

Managing Medical Debt: Strategies for Paying for Treatment

The financial burden of cancer treatment can be overwhelming, especially if your insurance doesn't cover all the costs. Medical debt can quickly add up, but there are steps you can take to manage these expenses.

Practical Tips:

- **Speak to the Hospital's Financial Department:** Many hospitals offer financial counseling or assistance programs to help patients pay their bills. Some may offer payment plans, sliding-scale fees, or other financial assistance options based on your income.

- **Negotiate with Providers:** Don't be afraid to negotiate with your healthcare providers for reduced rates, or ask if they have payment plans or assistance programs.

- **Consider Crowdfunding:** Some people choose to use crowdfunding platforms like GoFundMe to help with medical expenses. While this might not work for everyone, it can be an option to consider if you have a strong support network.

- **Explore Financial Aid and Charity Programs:** Look into national and local organizations that provide financial assistance to cancer patients. For example, foundations like the American Cancer Society may offer grants or direct financial assistance.

Estate Planning: Preparing for the Future

A cancer diagnosis often leads people to think about the future, especially when it comes to **estate planning** and ensuring that their wishes are met. Having these plans in place can reduce stress for both you and your loved ones.

Practical Tips:

- **Create or Update Your Will:** If you don't already have a will, consider creating one to outline how you want your assets to be distributed. If you already have a will, update it to reflect any changes in your life circumstances, such as a cancer diagnosis or changes in family relationships.

- **Power of Attorney:** A **durable power of attorney** allows you to designate someone to make financial and legal decisions on your behalf if you become unable to do so. This person can manage your bills, investments, and other legal matters if you're incapacitated.

- **Healthcare Proxy:** A **healthcare proxy** or **medical power of attorney** allows you to designate someone to make healthcare decisions for you if you're unable to make them yourself. This can include decisions about treatments, surgeries, and end-of-life care.

- **Living Will:** A **living will** is a document that specifies your preferences for medical treatments and end-of-life care, such as whether you want life-sustaining treatments in the event of a terminal illness. It can help ensure that your wishes are followed if you are unable to communicate them.

Life Insurance and Financial Planning: Ensuring Financial Security

Life insurance can provide financial security for your loved ones, but it's important to review your policy and ensure it meets your current needs. Cancer patients may also face challenges when applying for new life insurance policies, so understanding your options is key.

Practical Tips:

- **Review Your Life Insurance Policy:** Ensure your life insurance policy is up to date and reflects your current needs. If you already have a policy, make sure it includes sufficient coverage to support your family in case of your passing.

- **Consider Critical Illness Insurance:** Critical illness insurance is a type of policy that pays out a lump sum if you're diagnosed with a serious illness, such as cancer. If you don't have this type of coverage, you might want to consider it as a supplement to your existing insurance.

- **Consult a Financial Advisor:** A financial advisor can help you navigate the complexities of insurance, investments, and retirement planning. They can provide advice on managing medical costs and planning for the future, including tax strategies and saving for long-term care if necessary.

Taxes and Tax Relief: Understanding Your Tax Responsibilities and Benefits

Cancer treatment can impact your finances in various ways, including potential tax benefits. It's essential to understand how your diagnosis and treatment might affect your taxes.

Practical Tips:

- **Deduct Medical Expenses:** If your medical expenses are high, you may be eligible to deduct some of those expenses from your taxable income. The IRS allows individuals to deduct medical expenses that exceed 7.5% of their adjusted gross income (AGI). This can include costs for treatments, medications, travel to appointments, and more.

- **Check for Tax Credits:** Some states offer tax credits or financial assistance to cancer patients. Look into available programs in your area or ask your accountant about possible credits related to cancer treatment.

- **Tax-Free Cancer Benefits:** If you have a **critical illness insurance policy**, the payouts from the policy are typically tax-free. If you receive benefits from a cancer-related fundraiser, the funds may also be tax-free, but it's important to verify with a tax professional.

Legal Support and Advocacy: Understanding Your Rights

A cancer diagnosis can trigger a range of legal concerns, from employment discrimination to patient rights in healthcare. It's important to understand your legal rights and know when to seek professional help.

Practical Tips:

- **Know Your Rights:** If you're facing discrimination or difficulty accessing medical care, be aware of your rights under the **Americans with Disabilities Act (ADA)** and the **Family and Medical Leave Act (FMLA)**. Cancer patients are entitled to workplace accommodations and leave under these laws.

- **Seek Legal Aid:** If you're having trouble navigating insurance claims or if you believe your rights have been violated, consider consulting a **patient advocate** or **attorney** who specializes in cancer-related legal issues.

- **Join Advocacy Groups:** Cancer advocacy organizations can provide resources and support for legal and financial issues related to your diagnosis. Many of these organizations also offer free legal consultations for cancer patients.

Chapter 11: Supporting a Loved One with Breast Cancer

How to Be There for Someone

Supporting a loved one who is going through breast cancer can be one of the most meaningful things you can do, but it can also feel overwhelming. Every person's journey is unique, and they may have different needs at different times. Offering the right kind of help—emotionally, physically, and logistically—can make a world of difference. Here are some practical tips on how to be there for someone you care about during this challenging time.

Emotional Support: Be Present and Listen

One of the most important things you can do is to be there for your loved one, emotionally. People with breast cancer often experience a rollercoaster of emotions—fear, anger, sadness, and even guilt. Your role is to provide comfort and understanding.

- **Be a good listener:** Sometimes, what they need most is someone who can listen without judgment or interruption. Let them express their feelings, whether they want to talk about their diagnosis, their fears for the future, or even everyday life.

- **Acknowledge their emotions:** Cancer can stir up a mix of emotions, and it's important to validate their feelings. Say things like, "I can't imagine how hard this must be for you," or "It's okay to feel scared."

- **Offer reassurance, but be honest:** While it's important to stay positive, avoid offering empty platitudes like, "You'll be fine." Instead, offer genuine encouragement and support, acknowledging the difficulties they face while maintaining a hopeful outlook.

Physical Support: Offer Practical Help

Physical support can involve both direct assistance with daily tasks and ensuring they are comfortable and well-cared for.

- **Offer transportation to appointments:** Cancer treatments like chemotherapy, radiation, or surgeries can make it difficult for someone to drive. Offering rides to and from appointments can relieve them of stress and allow them to focus on their recovery.

- **Help with household tasks:** From grocery shopping to cleaning or cooking, offering a helping hand with household chores can be a huge relief. Ask if they need help with things like laundry, cleaning, or picking up medications, and don't be afraid to step in with specific offers rather than just saying, "Let me know if you need anything."

- **Provide physical comfort:** Simple acts like offering a warm blanket, a hand to hold during treatments, or a pillow for extra comfort can show your support in small but powerful ways. Physical touch can provide reassurance and ease anxiety.

Logistical Support: Organize the Practicalities

Cancer treatment can require a lot of logistical planning. Your loved one may be too tired or overwhelmed to manage the various aspects of treatment, recovery, and daily life. You can help by taking over some of the organizational tasks.

- **Help manage medical information:** Cancer treatment involves a lot of paperwork, doctor's visits, test results, and appointment scheduling. You can help by keeping track of appointments, medication schedules, and other important information. Offer to attend appointments with them if they'd like support in understanding what the doctors are saying.

- **Coordinate support networks:** Often, friends and family want to help but don't know how. Take the lead by organizing a meal train, setting up a calendar for visitors, or coordinating who will take them to their next appointment.

- **Help with finances:** Medical costs, insurance forms, and co-pays can add up quickly. If you're close enough, offer to help with understanding insurance policies, submitting claims, or even researching financial assistance options. This can be a huge weight off their shoulders.

Encourage Self-Care and Normalcy

Cancer treatment can make people feel isolated or disconnected from their usual lives. Encouraging your loved one to take time for themselves, or to maintain some level of normalcy, is essential for their mental health and recovery.

- **Encourage gentle activities:** Encourage them to rest when needed, but also suggest light activities like a walk in the park or watching a favorite movie. If they feel well enough, help them find small joys or engage in activities they love. This could be anything from reading a book together to doing a craft project.

- **Respect their boundaries:** Sometimes, they may not feel like socializing or talking about cancer. Respect their wishes and be patient. Don't push them into doing something they're not ready for.
- **Help them maintain their identity:** Cancer can make people feel as though they've lost their sense of self. Remind them of who they are beyond their diagnosis. Compliment their strengths, remind them of past achievements, and help them feel like themselves again.

Be Mindful of Your Own Well-Being

Supporting someone with cancer can be emotionally and physically draining. It's essential to care for yourself as well, so you can continue to provide the best support possible.

- **Don't neglect your own needs:** While it's natural to want to care for your loved one, it's also important to take breaks, practice self-care, and reach out for support when you need it.
- **Seek support for yourself:** If you feel overwhelmed, consider joining a support group for caregivers or talking to a counselor. It's okay to lean on others to help you navigate this challenging time.
- **Communicate openly with your loved one:** Let them know if you need to take a break or ask for help. Being honest about your own emotional needs can strengthen your relationship and prevent burnout.

Offer Encouragement without Pressure

During their treatment, your loved one might face setbacks, feel unmotivated, or lose hope. It's important to offer words of encouragement, but be careful not to pressure them into feeling a certain way.

- **Let them take the lead:** Sometimes, they may want to talk about their treatment or the future, and other times, they may just need a distraction. Follow their lead and don't push them into conversations they're not ready for.

- **Validate their experience:** Instead of offering advice or quick fixes, simply acknowledge their feelings. Phrases like "I'm here for you, no matter what," or "This is tough, but you're not alone," can be incredibly comforting.

Celebrate Milestones Together

Survivorship is filled with both challenges and triumphs. Celebrate the small victories, whether it's completing a round of chemotherapy, reaching the end of radiation, or simply getting through a tough day.

- **Mark milestones:** Whether it's a "chemo-free" day, finishing a difficult treatment cycle, or simply achieving a personal goal, celebrate these milestones. Small gestures like sending a congratulatory card, taking them out for a treat, or simply saying "You did it!" can go a long way in lifting their spirits.

- **Create positive memories:** Although treatment is hard, try to create moments of joy and laughter. Plan something special, whether it's a quiet evening at home, a trip to a favorite place, or a dinner with close friends to mark an important day in their journey.

Understanding the Treatment Process

Breast cancer treatment can be a complex, challenging, and sometimes overwhelming process for both the patient and their loved ones. As someone close to a person undergoing treatment, it's essential to understand what they're going through, not just physically, but emotionally and mentally as well. By gaining a deeper understanding of the treatment process, you can provide more effective support and help your loved one feel less isolated.

The Beginning of Treatment: Emotional and Mental Adjustments

When a loved one is first diagnosed with breast cancer, it's a life-altering moment, and the journey ahead often starts with a whirlwind of emotions. It's essential to recognize that the emotional toll of a breast cancer diagnosis can be just as overwhelming as the physical challenges of treatment. Here's how to support them:

- **Initial Reactions:** The first few weeks after a diagnosis can be filled with fear, confusion, and uncertainty. Many patients will feel overwhelmed by their new reality and all the medical information they suddenly need to process. It's important to offer emotional support without pushing for immediate action or decisions.

- **Mental Health Considerations:** Breast cancer patients often experience anxiety, depression, and stress. While it's important to stay positive, you should avoid forcing optimism. Sometimes, simply acknowledging how hard things are can make them feel heard and understood. Offer a safe space where they can express their feelings.

The Treatment Plan: What to Expect

Breast cancer treatment is highly individualized. The plan depends on factors like the type and stage of cancer, the patient's overall health, and personal preferences. Treatment may involve one or more therapies, including surgery, chemotherapy, radiation, and targeted therapies. Understanding each step of the process helps you provide meaningful support.

- **Surgery:** The first step for many people with breast cancer is surgery, either a lumpectomy (removal of the tumor) or a mastectomy (removal of one or both breasts). This may also include the removal of nearby lymph nodes. Surgery can have a significant emotional impact, as the patient may feel a loss of identity or concern about how they will look post-surgery. Be supportive during recovery, as they may need help with mobility or basic daily tasks.

- **Chemotherapy:** Chemotherapy is often used to kill cancer cells or shrink tumors before surgery. It's a system-wide treatment that affects the entire body, and it can cause significant side effects like nausea, fatigue, hair loss, and weakened immune function. Your loved one may experience physical changes, and it's important to offer comfort and understanding as they navigate these difficult times. Encourage rest and help manage side effects by providing nutritious meals, helping with chores, or simply sitting with them during treatments.

- **Radiation Therapy:** After surgery, many patients undergo radiation therapy, which uses high-energy rays to target and kill remaining cancer cells. Radiation is typically localized to the breast or chest area, but it can cause fatigue, skin irritation, and changes in mood. Your support during this phase can help them feel less anxious and more comfortable, as radiation treatments often last several weeks. Be mindful that they may feel physically drained, so offering practical help like running errands or preparing meals can be invaluable.

- **Targeted Therapies and Hormone Therapy:** If the cancer is hormone receptor-positive or HER2-positive, your loved one may undergo targeted therapy or hormone therapy. These treatments work to block specific proteins or hormones that contribute to cancer growth. While these treatments are generally less physically taxing than chemotherapy, they may still cause fatigue, hot flashes, or other symptoms. Understanding the specific type of treatment your loved one is undergoing can help you anticipate their needs and offer the right support.

The Physical Impact of Treatment: How to Lend a Hand

Breast cancer treatment can take a toll on a person's body. While some side effects are temporary, others may last longer, requiring both physical and emotional support. Here are some ways you can help them manage:

- **Fatigue:** One of the most common side effects of cancer treatment is fatigue. It's not just being tired—it's an overwhelming exhaustion that rest alone can't fix. Your loved one may feel wiped out for weeks or months. Offer to help with tasks, provide opportunities to rest, and avoid scheduling too many activities that could overwhelm them.

- **Nausea and Appetite Changes:** Chemotherapy can cause nausea, loss of appetite, and weight changes. Help your loved one by preparing or bringing meals that are easy to digest and high in nutrients. Make sure they stay hydrated and encourage them to eat smaller, more frequent meals if they have trouble with larger portions.

- **Physical Care and Hygiene:** Depending on the type of surgery, your loved one may have wounds that need special care, or they may need help with simple activities like bathing, dressing, or walking. Be gentle and patient, and provide assistance without making them feel like a burden.

Managing Emotional and Mental Health During Treatment

In addition to physical symptoms, breast cancer treatment can also lead to emotional and psychological challenges. Helping your loved one maintain their mental health is crucial to their overall well-being.

- **Addressing Body Image Issues:** Many women struggle with body image concerns, especially after surgery, chemotherapy, or radiation. Some may experience changes in their appearance, including hair loss, weight changes, or surgical scars. Be sensitive to their feelings about their body and offer positive affirmations about their strength, beauty, and resilience.

- **Social Support and Interaction:** While they might want to rest or have some time alone, don't let them feel isolated. Encourage visits from close friends and family members, and consider organizing small social activities or outings that they can handle.

However, be mindful not to overwhelm them—always check in to ensure they feel up to engaging.

- **Mental Health Resources:** Encourage your loved one to talk to a counselor, support groups, or mental health professionals. Many hospitals offer psychological support or cancer-specific counseling, which can be an invaluable resource during the treatment process.

Ongoing Adjustments: Helping with Life After Treatment

Once the active phase of treatment ends, many breast cancer survivors face a new set of challenges, such as dealing with the fear of recurrence, managing long-term side effects, and adjusting back to their "new normal." Here's how you can continue supporting them:

- **Post-Treatment Fatigue:** After treatment, it's common for patients to continue feeling fatigued or to experience a lack of energy. Offer continued emotional support, and help them manage day-to-day tasks as they recover and regain strength.

- **Survivorship Care Plans:** Many survivors will be given a survivorship care plan, which includes guidelines for ongoing monitoring and follow-up appointments. Assist them in scheduling these visits or helping track medications or treatments, especially as the patient adjusts to a less frequent medical regimen.

- **Help Manage Recurrence Anxiety:** The fear of recurrence can linger even after treatment ends. Being there to listen, encourage, and reassure them during this time is essential. Remind them that they are not alone in this and that there are resources available to help them cope with this fear.

Caring for the Caregiver

Caregiving is often seen as an act of love and devotion, but it can take a significant emotional, mental, and physical toll on those who provide support to breast cancer patients. Caregivers often prioritize their loved one's needs over their own, leading to burnout, stress, and sometimes physical health issues. It's crucial to recognize that caregivers need care too, and finding a balance between supporting the patient and looking after themselves is vital for both their well-being and the patient's recovery.

The Emotional Toll of Caregiving

Being a caregiver for someone undergoing breast cancer treatment can be an emotional rollercoaster. You might feel a mix of anxiety, sadness, frustration, and helplessness as you witness the physical and emotional challenges your loved one faces. At the same time, the responsibility of being their primary source of support can create pressure and stress.

- **Feelings of Helplessness:** It's common for caregivers to feel helpless when they see their loved one in pain or struggling with treatment side effects. The desire to "fix" things can lead to frustration when things are out of your control.

- **Fear and Anxiety:** Caregivers often share in the fear and uncertainty about the future. Worrying about the patient's health, treatment outcomes, and long-term prognosis can be overwhelming. It's natural to feel anxious, but it's important to recognize that these feelings are valid and to take steps to manage them.

- **Guilt:** Many caregivers feel guilty about taking time for themselves or feel like they aren't doing enough.

This guilt can be compounded by seeing the patient's emotional or physical distress. However, remember that self-care is essential to being an effective caregiver, and taking breaks doesn't mean you love or care any less.

The Physical Toll of Caregiving

Caregivers often neglect their own physical health while tending to the patient's needs. The constant demands of caregiving—whether it's managing medical appointments, helping with daily tasks, or providing emotional support—can result in physical exhaustion.

- **Fatigue:** The emotional strain and long hours spent caring for a loved one can lead to caregiver fatigue, where you feel drained both physically and mentally. Exhaustion can make it difficult to be present for the patient and can even impact your own health.

- **Sleep Deprivation:** Caring for someone with breast cancer may mean late nights spent at medical appointments or worrying about their condition. Sleep disturbances, either from staying up late or being hyper-alert, can lead to long-term health problems like weakened immunity, poor concentration, and physical fatigue.

- **Physical Health Issues:** Caregivers may face their own physical health challenges, such as back pain from helping the patient move, lifting heavy objects, or spending hours at the hospital. The stress of caregiving can also contribute to headaches, digestive issues, or weight fluctuations.

Ways to Find Balance and Care for Yourself

To provide the best support to your loved one, it's essential to maintain your own well-being. Here are some strategies for caregivers to find balance and avoid burnout:

A. Set Boundaries and Prioritize Self-Care

- **Schedule Time for Yourself:** It's crucial to set aside time each day or week for activities that recharge you. Whether it's taking a walk, reading a book, or enjoying a hobby, find something that brings you joy and relaxation. Even 15-30 minutes a day can make a big difference.

- **Take Breaks When Needed:** Caregiving doesn't mean you have to be on-call 24/7. Take breaks to step away from caregiving responsibilities. This could mean asking a friend or family member to step in for a few hours, or utilizing respite care services to give you time to rest and recover.

- **Delegate Tasks:** Don't be afraid to ask for help. Family, friends, or even community organizations may be willing to assist with chores, running errands, or offering emotional support. By sharing the load, you can reduce stress and focus on what's most important.

B. Seek Emotional Support

- **Talk to Someone:** Whether it's a friend, a counselor, or a support group, talking to someone who understands your experience can be incredibly therapeutic. Expressing your feelings and frustrations can help release emotional tension and prevent bottling up negative emotions.

- **Join a Caregiver Support Group:** Many cancer organizations offer support groups specifically for caregivers. These groups provide a safe space to share your struggles, connect with others in similar situations, and gain advice on managing stress.

- **Practice Mindfulness:** Techniques like meditation, yoga, and deep breathing exercises can help reduce stress and improve emotional resilience. Mindfulness helps caregivers stay present in the moment and reduces anxiety about the future.

C. Maintain Physical Health

- **Exercise Regularly:** Physical activity is an excellent way to manage stress and boost energy levels. Even a short daily walk, stretching, or yoga session can improve your mood, increase stamina, and help you feel better physically and emotionally.

- **Eat a Balanced Diet:** Caregivers often skip meals or eat poorly when they're overwhelmed, but good nutrition is essential for maintaining energy and overall health. Try to focus on eating nutrient-dense foods, and when possible, involve your loved one in meal planning or cooking to make it a shared activity.

- **Rest and Sleep:** While it can be difficult, it's essential to prioritize rest. Sleep is a major contributor to physical health and emotional stability. If sleep disruptions are a problem, try to set a bedtime routine or use relaxation techniques to help you unwind.

D. Stay Organized and Plan Ahead

- **Create a Caregiving Schedule:** Juggling medical appointments, treatments, and daily caregiving tasks can feel overwhelming. Keep track of appointments, medication schedules, and other responsibilities by creating a daily or weekly plan. Use a calendar, app, or notebook to stay organized and minimize stress.

- **Know Your Limits:** It's important to recognize when you're reaching your limits. If you feel overwhelmed or are getting sick, it's okay to ask for help. Caregiving is a team effort, and you are not alone in this.

Know When to Seek Help

It's important to remember that you don't have to be the sole caregiver, and it's okay to ask for help when needed. Seeking support for yourself is not a sign of weakness; rather, it's a sign of strength and an essential step in being able to provide the best care for your loved one.

- **Professional Help:** If you're feeling physically or emotionally drained, consider speaking with a therapist or counselor who can offer support and coping strategies. Many therapists specialize in helping caregivers navigate the challenges of chronic illness and can provide tools to prevent burnout.

- **Respite Care:** Many healthcare providers or cancer centers offer respite care, where professionals come in to assist with care duties for a set period. This allows caregivers to take a break while ensuring that their loved one is still receiving the necessary care.

- **Community Resources:** Check with local cancer organizations or support groups for additional resources, including financial assistance, respite care, or meal delivery services. Many organizations are specifically designed to support both the patient and the caregiver throughout the cancer journey.

Conclusion

Key Takeaways

Breast cancer is a complex disease with many layers, but understanding it is essential for prevention, early detection, and effective treatment. Here's a summary of the most important points from each chapter to help you navigate this important topic:

What Is Breast Cancer?

Breast cancer is the uncontrolled growth of abnormal cells in the breast, which can form a lump or tumor. These cancerous cells can spread to other parts of the body. Understanding the types of cells involved and how breast cancer develops in the body is key to recognizing its complexity.

Types of Breast Cancer

There are different types of breast cancer, with **invasive ductal carcinoma (IDC)** being the most common. Other types include **invasive lobular carcinoma (ILC)**, **inflammatory breast cancer**, and **triple-negative breast cancer**. The subtype affects treatment decisions and prognosis.

Risk Factors

Breast cancer risk is influenced by genetic factors like mutations in **BRCA1 and BRCA2**, hormonal influences such as early menstruation and late menopause, lifestyle factors like alcohol use, smoking, and obesity, and environmental exposures to toxins. Understanding these risks can help guide prevention strategies.

Myths vs. Facts

It's important to dispel common misconceptions about breast cancer. For example, while breast cancer can affect anyone, it does not only affect older women. Early detection and awareness of risk factors can help dispel these myths and improve outcomes.

Tumor Development

Breast cancer grows when cells divide uncontrollably, creating tumors. Cancer cells can spread (metastasize) to other parts of the body, affecting distant organs. The process of metastasis is crucial in understanding how the disease progresses and how it's treated.

Molecular Subtypes

Molecular subtypes, such as **HER2-positive** and **hormone receptor-positive** cancers, are defined by specific markers that affect how the cancer behaves. These subtypes guide personalized treatment options, such as targeted therapies or hormone therapy.

Genetic Mutations and Heredity

Mutations in genes like **BRCA1** and **BRCA2** significantly increase the risk of developing breast cancer. Genetic testing helps identify individuals who may benefit from preventive measures, such as mastectomies or early screening.

Lifestyle Factors

Diet, exercise, alcohol consumption, and tobacco use all play roles in breast cancer risk. Maintaining a healthy weight, regular exercise, and limiting alcohol intake can help reduce your overall risk.

Breastfeeding

Breastfeeding has been shown to reduce the risk of breast cancer, possibly due to hormonal changes that occur during breastfeeding and the shedding of breast tissue cells.

Hormonal Therapy and Birth Control

Hormonal contraceptives and hormone replacement therapy may increase breast cancer risk in some women. Understanding these treatments and discussing alternatives with your doctor is essential in risk assessment and prevention strategies.

Genetic Testing

Genetic testing, particularly for **BRCA mutations**, allows for early detection and intervention. Those at high genetic risk can benefit from increased surveillance or preventive treatments, which can significantly reduce their risk of developing breast cancer.

Environmental Factors

Exposure to environmental toxins, such as certain chemicals and radiation, may increase the risk of breast cancer. Reducing exposure to known carcinogens and making informed lifestyle choices can help minimize this risk.

Screening Methods

Regular screenings are vital for early detection of breast cancer. **Mammograms**, **ultrasound**, and **MRI** are essential tools for identifying abnormalities. Each method has its role, and the choice of which test to use depends on age, risk factors, and other variables.

Self-Examination

Performing breast self-exams is a valuable tool for noticing changes in the breast. While it shouldn't replace clinical screenings, it empowers individuals to be proactive about their health and seek medical attention if changes are noticed.

Signs and Symptoms

Common signs of breast cancer include lumps, changes in the size or shape of the breast, and nipple discharge. Less common symptoms can include pain or swelling. Early detection is crucial, so it's important to pay attention to your body and consult a healthcare provider if you notice any changes.

The Diagnostic Process

Breast cancer diagnosis involves imaging (mammograms, ultrasound, MRI) and testing (biopsy). Doctors will use these to assess the tumor's size, location, and stage, helping to form a personalized treatment plan.

Understanding Staging

Staging breast cancer (Stage 0 to Stage IV) is essential to understanding the severity of the disease and the prognosis. The stage reflects how far the cancer has spread, with Stage 0 being localized and Stage IV indicating widespread metastasis.

Lymph Node Involvement

Lymph node involvement plays a significant role in staging and prognosis. Cancer cells in lymph nodes indicate that the cancer has begun to spread, which may affect treatment decisions and outcomes.

Prognostic Factors

Factors such as tumor grade, receptor status, and overall health influence the outcome of breast cancer treatment. Lower-grade tumors and favorable receptor status often result in better outcomes.

The Role of Molecular Testing

Molecular tests can help predict how aggressive a breast cancer is and guide treatment decisions. Testing can identify targetable genetic mutations, such as **HER2-positive** cancers, allowing for more effective and individualized treatments.

Treatment Options: Surgery, Radiation, Chemotherapy

Breast cancer treatment can include **surgery** (lumpectomy or mastectomy), **radiation therapy**, and **chemotherapy**. Each approach has its role in removing or shrinking tumors, preventing recurrence, and managing side effects.

Targeted Therapies and Immunotherapy

Newer treatments, such as **targeted therapies** and **immunotherapy**, focus on attacking specific cancer cells or boosting the immune system to fight cancer. These treatments are increasingly becoming part of personalized care plans.

Hormone Therapy

Hormone therapies are used for **hormone receptor-positive** cancers, blocking estrogen or progesterone to prevent cancer growth. These treatments can be taken as pills or injections and are an important tool for long-term management.

Clinical Trials

Clinical trials offer patients access to the latest treatments and therapies. Participating in a clinical trial can help advance cancer research and provide opportunities for innovative treatments not yet widely available.

Emotional and Psychological Impact

A breast cancer diagnosis affects both the patient and their loved ones emotionally. Feelings of anxiety, depression, and body image concerns are common. Seeking support from professionals, support groups, or loved ones can help manage these challenges.

Survivorship and Life After Treatment

Life after treatment involves ongoing monitoring, managing the fear of recurrence, and maintaining a healthy lifestyle. Many survivors thrive post-treatment by focusing on their emotional and physical well-being and celebrating their journey.

Long-Term Follow-Up and Quality of Life

Regular follow-ups are essential to catch recurrences early. Survivors can improve their quality of life through managing fatigue, sleep, relationships, and finding joy in their post-treatment life.

Legal and Financial Considerations

Understanding the legal and financial aspects of breast cancer—such as insurance, work, and disability—can ease the burden. Resources like financial assistance and legal support are available to help navigate these challenges.

Hope and Future Outlook

The journey through breast cancer is undoubtedly challenging, but the future holds a world of hope. Ongoing research continues to unlock new discoveries and treatments that are changing the landscape of breast cancer care. From personalized medicine to breakthrough immunotherapies, the fight against breast cancer has never been more promising.

Every year, scientists make significant strides in understanding the disease at a molecular level, leading to more effective treatments and better outcomes for patients. New technologies, like liquid biopsies and advanced genetic testing, are making it possible to detect cancer earlier and with greater precision. The ability to tailor treatments to the unique genetic makeup of each patient is revolutionizing cancer care, making therapies more effective and less toxic.

Thanks to advancements in treatments such as **targeted therapies**, **immunotherapies**, and **hormone treatments**, survival rates have been steadily improving. The focus on personalized care means that more patients are receiving the right treatments for their specific type of cancer, and new drugs and therapies continue to be developed to target cancer cells with greater accuracy.

Additionally, cancer prevention and early detection efforts have made great strides. Advances in screening methods and awareness have led to earlier diagnoses, which are key to improving survival rates. Moreover, the development of **preventive medications** and interventions for high-risk individuals is offering hope to those at higher risk of developing breast cancer.

In terms of survivorship, life after treatment has evolved as well. With improved recovery options, psychological support, and rehabilitation programs, many breast cancer survivors go on to live full, active, and meaningful lives. The emphasis on **quality of life**, long-term care, and emotional well-being ensures that patients not only survive but thrive in the years after their diagnosis.

The future is bright, and the outlook for breast cancer patients continues to improve. With the global community of researchers, healthcare providers, and advocates working together, the goal of finding a cure and providing better, more effective treatment options is within reach. No matter the stage of breast cancer, the spirit of hope, resilience, and progress shines brightly.

As we look to the future, one thing is certain: breast cancer is no longer the insurmountable challenge it once seemed. With continued research, improved treatments, and the power of hope, breast cancer patients are not only surviving—they are thriving, and more will continue to do so every year.

Glossary of Medical Terms

Here is a glossary of commonly used medical terms related to breast cancer, which can help clarify the technical language and jargon used throughout this book.

Adenocarcinoma

A type of cancer that begins in the cells of a gland, such as the cells lining the ducts or lobes of the breast.

Biopsy

A medical test in which a small sample of tissue is removed from the body for examination under a microscope to determine if it is cancerous.

BRCA1 and BRCA2

Genes that help repair DNA. Mutations in these genes significantly increase the risk of breast cancer and other cancers.

Chemotherapy

A type of cancer treatment that uses drugs to kill cancer cells or stop their growth. Chemotherapy can be given orally or intravenously.

Ductal Carcinoma in Situ (DCIS)

A non-invasive form of breast cancer where abnormal cells are found in the milk ducts but have not spread outside the ducts.

Estrogen Receptor (ER)-Positive

A type of breast cancer where the cancer cells have receptors for estrogen, which can fuel the growth of the cancer. Hormone therapy is often used to treat ER-positive breast cancer.

HER2-Positive

A type of breast cancer where the cancer cells have higher-than-normal levels of the HER2 protein, which promotes cancer cell growth. Targeted therapies can be used to treat HER2-positive cancer.

Invasive (Infiltrating) Ductal Carcinoma (IDC)

The most common type of breast cancer, IDC starts in the milk ducts and spreads to surrounding tissue.

Invasive Lobular Carcinoma (ILC)

A type of breast cancer that begins in the milk-producing lobules and spreads to surrounding tissue. It is the second most common type of breast cancer.

Lymph Nodes

Small, bean-shaped structures that are part of the lymphatic system, which helps fight infections. Cancer can spread to lymph nodes, making them an important factor in staging breast cancer.

Lymphedema

Swelling that occurs when lymph fluid builds up in the body, often in the arms or legs, as a result of surgery or radiation treatment affecting the lymphatic system.

Lumpectomy

Surgical removal of a tumor from the breast while preserving the surrounding breast tissue.

Mastectomy

Surgical removal of the entire breast to treat or prevent breast cancer. There are different types, including total mastectomy and modified radical mastectomy.

Metastasis

The spread of cancer cells from the original (primary) site to other parts of the body. For example, breast cancer cells can spread to the lungs, bones, or liver.

MRI (Magnetic Resonance Imaging)

A non-invasive imaging technique that uses strong magnetic fields and radio waves to create detailed images of the inside of the body. It is sometimes used in breast cancer screening, especially for high-risk individuals.

Oncology

The branch of medicine that focuses on the diagnosis, treatment, and management of cancer.

Radiation Therapy

A cancer treatment that uses high-energy rays (such as X-rays) to target and kill cancer cells or shrink tumors.

Recurrence

When cancer returns after a period of remission. A recurrence can occur in the same location or in other parts of the body.

Receptor Status

Refers to the presence or absence of certain proteins on the surface of breast cancer cells, such as estrogen receptors (ER), progesterone receptors (PR), or HER2 receptors. This information helps determine treatment options.

Stage 0 to Stage IV

Breast cancer is staged based on its size, location, and whether it has spread.

Stage 0 is non-invasive (e.g., DCIS).

Stage I is early-stage cancer confined to the breast.

Stage II involves some spread to nearby lymph nodes.

Stage III involves extensive spread to lymph nodes or chest wall.

Stage IV is metastatic cancer, where the cancer has spread to distant parts of the body.

Tamoxifen

A medication used in the treatment of hormone receptor-positive breast cancer. It blocks the effects of estrogen, which can stimulate the growth of cancer cells.

Targeted Therapy

Cancer treatments that target specific molecules involved in cancer cell growth and survival. These therapies are often used for cancers that express certain proteins or genes, such as HER2-positive breast cancer.

Triple-Negative Breast Cancer (TNBC)

A type of breast cancer that does not have receptors for estrogen, progesterone, or HER2. It is often more aggressive and harder to treat than other types of breast cancer.

Tumor Grade

Refers to how abnormal the cancer cells look under a microscope. High-grade tumors tend to grow faster and are more aggressive, while low-grade tumors grow more slowly.

Tumor Markers

Substances found in the blood or tissue that can be used to help diagnose cancer, track its progression, or assess treatment effectiveness.

Ultrasound

A non-invasive imaging technique that uses sound waves to create images of the inside of the body. It is often used to examine suspicious breast lumps or cysts.

Women's Health Initiative (WHI)

A long-term national study focused on strategies to prevent diseases in women, including breast cancer. It has provided valuable data on hormone replacement therapy and its link to breast cancer risk.

Frequently Asked Questions (FAQs)

Here are answers to some of the most common questions people have about breast cancer and its treatment options.

What is breast cancer?

Breast cancer occurs when abnormal cells in the breast tissue begin to grow uncontrollably, forming a lump or mass. It can develop in various parts of the breast, such as the ducts (the milk-carrying tubes) or lobules (the milk-producing glands). These cancerous cells can spread to other parts of the body if left untreated.

What are the common symptoms of breast cancer?

Common symptoms of breast cancer include:

- A lump in the breast or underarm.
- Changes in the size, shape, or appearance of the breast.
- Unexplained pain in the breast or nipple.
- Nipple discharge that isn't breast milk.
- Skin changes like redness or puckering on the breast.

However, it's important to remember that not all breast lumps are cancerous, and these symptoms can also be caused by other conditions.

What are the risk factors for breast cancer?

Several factors can increase the risk of developing breast cancer, including:

- **Age**: The risk increases with age, particularly after 50.
- **Family history**: A family history of breast cancer, especially in first-degree relatives, can increase your risk.
- **Genetic mutations**: Mutations in genes like **BRCA1** and **BRCA2** increase the risk.
- **Hormonal factors**: Early menstruation, late menopause, and hormone replacement therapy (HRT) use can influence risk.
- **Lifestyle factors**: Poor diet, lack of exercise, smoking, and excessive alcohol consumption can also contribute.

How is breast cancer diagnosed?

Breast cancer is often diagnosed through a combination of methods, including:

- **Mammograms**: X-ray images of the breast used to detect abnormal changes.
- **Ultrasound**: Uses sound waves to create images of the breast and help distinguish between solid masses and cysts.
- **MRI (Magnetic Resonance Imaging)**: Provides detailed images of the breast and is sometimes used for high-risk individuals.
- **Biopsy**: A sample of tissue is taken from a suspicious area to check for cancer cells.

What are the different types of breast cancer?

There are several types of breast cancer, including:

- **Invasive Ductal Carcinoma (IDC)**: The most common type, starting in the milk ducts and spreading to other parts of the breast.

- **Invasive Lobular Carcinoma (ILC)**: Starts in the lobules (milk-producing glands) and can spread to other parts.

- **Inflammatory Breast Cancer (IBC)**: A rare and aggressive form where the breast becomes red, swollen, and warm.

- **Ductal Carcinoma In Situ (DCIS)**: A non-invasive, early form of cancer confined to the milk ducts.

- **Triple-negative breast cancer**: A form that lacks estrogen, progesterone, and HER2 receptors, making it harder to treat with targeted therapies.

What are the treatment options for breast cancer?

Treatment options vary based on the stage, type, and genetic makeup of the cancer but generally include:

- **Surgery**: Removing the tumor or whole breast (mastectomy).

- **Chemotherapy**: Drugs used to kill cancer cells or stop them from growing.

- **Radiation therapy**: High-energy rays used to target cancer cells after surgery.

- **Hormone therapy**: Drugs that block or lower hormones like estrogen to slow or stop the growth of hormone-receptor-positive breast cancers.

- **Targeted therapy**: Drugs that specifically target cancer cells without affecting healthy ones.

- **Immunotherapy**: Boosts the immune system to fight cancer cells.
- **Clinical trials**: New experimental treatments that may be offered as part of ongoing research.

What is the difference between a lumpectomy and a mastectomy?

- **Lumpectomy**: This is a breast-conserving surgery where only the tumor and a small margin of healthy tissue are removed. It's typically used for early-stage cancer.
- **Mastectomy**: Involves the removal of the entire breast. This is often recommended for larger tumors or when cancer has spread throughout the breast tissue.

What are the side effects of chemotherapy?

Chemotherapy can cause a variety of side effects, including:

- Fatigue
- Hair loss
- Nausea and vomiting
- Increased risk of infection
- Anemia (low red blood cell count)
- Changes in appetite
- Skin or nail changes

Many of these side effects are temporary, but they can vary depending on the drugs used.

What are hormone receptor-positive and HER2-positive breast cancers?

- **Hormone receptor-positive**: These breast cancers grow in response to hormones like estrogen or progesterone. They are often treated with hormone therapies to block the hormones that fuel tumor growth.

- **HER2-positive**: These cancers have higher than normal levels of the HER2 protein, which promotes cancer cell growth. Targeted therapies like Herceptin are used to block HER2 and slow tumor growth.

Can breast cancer be prevented?

While there's no guaranteed way to prevent breast cancer, there are steps you can take to lower your risk:

- Maintain a healthy weight, exercise regularly, and eat a balanced diet.
- Limit alcohol consumption and avoid tobacco use.
- Consider genetic testing if you have a family history of breast cancer.
- Breastfeed, if possible, as breastfeeding may reduce the risk.
- Talk to your doctor about medications or treatments if you are at high risk (e.g., Tamoxifen or mastectomy for high-risk individuals).

How do I cope emotionally with a breast cancer diagnosis?

Being diagnosed with breast cancer can be overwhelming. Here are some strategies to cope emotionally:

- Lean on your support system—family, friends, and support groups.
- Consider speaking with a counselor or therapist to address feelings of fear, anxiety, or depression.
- Practice mindfulness and relaxation techniques to manage stress.
- Stay informed and take an active role in your treatment decisions.

What is the prognosis for breast cancer?

The prognosis for breast cancer depends on several factors, including the stage at diagnosis, the type of cancer, the size of the tumor, and whether the cancer has spread. In general:

- Early-stage breast cancer has a much better prognosis than advanced stages.
- Hormone receptor-positive and HER2-positive cancers often have more favorable outcomes with targeted therapies.

What is the role of clinical trials in breast cancer treatment?

Clinical trials play a key role in advancing breast cancer treatment. They test new therapies, drugs, or treatment combinations that might offer better results than current standard treatments. Participating in a clinical trial could provide access to cutting-edge therapies, though it's important to discuss the potential risks and benefits with your healthcare team.

What can I expect after completing treatment?

After treatment, patients are often monitored through regular follow-up appointments, including physical exams, imaging tests, and blood tests to detect any recurrence. Many survivors also experience "survivorship issues," such as managing side effects or coping with the emotional impact of cancer. It's important to have a plan for long-term care and to remain vigilant for any changes in your body.

Resources for Information and Support

For those seeking more information or support during their journey with breast cancer, there are numerous organizations, websites, and resources that can provide valuable guidance, assistance, and community. Below is a curated list to help you find the support you need:

National and International Organizations

1. **American Cancer Society (ACS)**
    - Website: www.cancer.org
    - Offers comprehensive information on breast cancer, treatment options, emotional support, and resources for patients and caregivers.

2. **Breast Cancer Research Foundation (BCRF)**
    - Website: www.bcrf.org
    - Focuses on funding innovative breast cancer research and providing resources for patients.

3. **Susan G. Komen Foundation**
    - Website: www.komen.org
    - A leading breast cancer organization, offering support, education, and funding for breast cancer research.

4. **National Breast Cancer Foundation (NBCF)**
    - Website: www.nationalbreastcancer.org
    - Provides education, support, and early detection services for breast cancer patients.

5. **Breast Cancer Care (UK)**
   - Website: www.breastcancercare.org.uk
   - Offers support services, information on diagnosis, treatment, and living with breast cancer.

6. **CancerCare**
   - Website: www.cancercare.org
   - Provides free counseling, support groups, and financial assistance for cancer patients and families.

7. **Living Beyond Breast Cancer (LBBC)**
   - Website: www.lbbc.org
   - Offers support and education to individuals affected by breast cancer at all stages of their diagnosis and treatment.

8. **International Agency for Research on Cancer (IARC)**
   - Website: www.iarc.who.int
   - A global resource providing scientific data on cancer prevention, including information on breast cancer.

Online Resources and Communities

1. **Breastcancer.org**
   - Website: www.breastcancer.org
   - A reliable online resource offering in-depth information on breast cancer diagnosis, treatment, coping, and support.

2. **Smart Patients**
   - Website: www.smartpatients.com

- An online community for patients with cancer to share experiences, discuss treatments, and find support.

3. **MyBreastCancerTeam**
    - Website: www.mybreastcancerteam.com
    - A social network for individuals affected by breast cancer to connect, share, and support one another.

4. **Cancer Support Community**
    - Website: www.cancersupportcommunity.org
    - Offers free online and in-person support groups, wellness programs, and information on navigating cancer.

Support Hotlines and Counseling Services

1. **National Cancer Institute (NCI) Cancer Information Service**
    - Phone: 1-800-4-CANCER (1-800-422-6237)
    - Website: www.cancer.gov
    - Offers free, confidential information about cancer, clinical trials, and other resources.

2. **American Cancer Society Helpline**
    - Phone: 1-800-227-2345
    - Website: www.cancer.org
    - Provides information and support to anyone facing cancer, including counseling and referrals.

3. **CancerCare Helpline**

- Phone: 1-800-813-HOPE (1-800-813-4673)
- Website: www.cancercare.org
- Provides free professional counseling and support services for people living with cancer.

Books for Patients and Caregivers

1. *The Breast Cancer Survival Manual* by John Link, M.D.
    - A comprehensive guide for patients navigating diagnosis and treatment.
2. *Breast Cancer: The Complete Guide* by Robert A. Wise and Lisa A. Weisberg
    - A thorough resource for breast cancer patients and families covering everything from prevention to recovery.
3. *The New Era of Breast Cancer* by Susan M. Love, M.D.
    - Dr. Susan Love explores the latest breakthroughs in breast cancer research and treatment options.
4. *Cancer Recovery Nutrition* by Walter C. Willett
    - Offers dietary recommendations for cancer patients, with a focus on recovery and maintaining health after treatment.

Helpful Mobile Apps

1. **MyCancerHome**
    - An app designed to provide cancer patients with information on their diagnosis and treatments, including clinical trials.

2. **CancerCare**
    - Offers access to emotional support, educational resources, and online support groups for cancer patients.

Other Resources

- **Genetic Testing Resources**: Talk to your doctor about options for genetic testing such as BRCA testing. You can also visit www.brcaexchange.org for more information.

- **Financial Assistance Programs**: Some organizations offer financial help for cancer-related costs. The **Cancer Financial Assistance Coalition (CFAC)** is a great starting point: www.cancerfac.org.

Printed in Great Britain
by Amazon